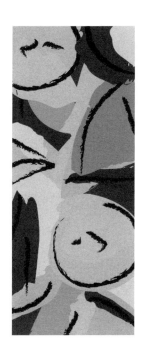

MacArthur-Bates Communicative Development Inventories

User's Guide and Technical Manual

SECOND EDITION

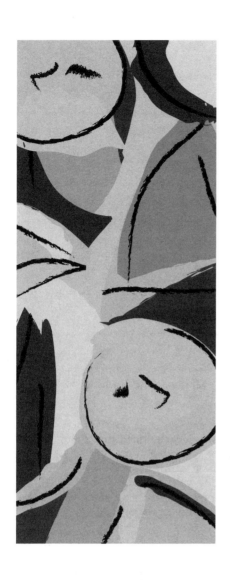

MacArthur-Bates Communicative Development Inventories

User's Guide and
Technical Manual

SECOND EDITION

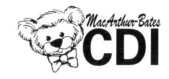

by

Larry Fenson, Ph.D.

Virginia A. Marchman, Ph.D.

Donna J. Thal, Ph.D.

Philip S. Dale, Ph.D.

J. Steven Reznick, Ph.D.

Elizabeth Bates, Ph.D.

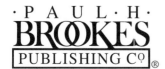

·P·A·U·L·H·
BROOKES
PUBLISHING CO.®

Baltimore • London • Sydney

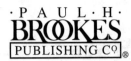

Paul H. Brookes Publishing Co.
Post Office Box 10624
Baltimore, Maryland 21285-0624

www.brookespublishing.com

Typeset by Integrated Publishing Solutions, Grand Rapids, Michigan.
Manufactured in the United States of America by
Versa Press, Inc., East Peoria, Illinois.

To learn more about the MacArthur-Bates Communicative Development Inventories
(CDIs), go to www.brookespublishing.com.

This manual accompanies the MacArthur-Bates Communicative Development Inventories (CDIs), which may be purchased in packages of machine-scannable forms or desktop-scannable forms. Desktop-scannable versions of the MacArthur-Bates Communicative Development Inventory–III (CDI-III) are available as well. In addition, the *MacArthur Inventarios del Desarrollo de Habilidades Comunicativas: User's Guide and Technical Manual* and machine- and desktop-scannable versions of the Spanish forms are available. To order, contact Paul H. Brookes Publishing Co. (1-800-638-3775; 410-337-9580; custserv@brookespublishing.com).

Library of Congress Cataloging-in-Publication Data

Fenson, Larry.
    MacArthur-Bates Communicative Development Inventories: user's guide and technical manual / by Larry Fenson . . . [et al.]. — 2nd ed.
        p.   cm.
    Includes bibliographical references and index.
    ISBN-13: 978-1-55766-884-4 (pbk.)
    ISBN-10: 1-55766-884-1 (pbk.)
    1. Language acquisition—Ability testing—Handbooks, manuals, etc.   2. Nonverbal communication in children—Ability testing—Handbooks, manuals, etc.   I. Title.
P118.P43 2006
418.0076—dc22   2006015997

British Library Cataloguing in Publication data are available from the British Library.

CONTENTS

LIST OF TABLES AND FIGURES

THE CDI ADVISORY BOARD

Chair, **Larry Fenson, Ph.D.**
Department of Psychology
San Diego State University
lfenson@sunstroke.sdsu.edu

Philip S. Dale, Ph.D.
Department of Speech and Hearing
  Sciences
The University of New Mexico
dalep@unm.edu

Donna Jackson-Maldonado, Ph.D.
Facultad de Lenguas y Letras
[Department of Languages and Literature]
University Autónoma de Querétaro
Mexico
djackson@uaq.mx

Virginia A. Marchman, Ph.D.
Department of Psychology
Stanford University
marchman@psych.stanford.edu

J. Steven Reznick, Ph.D.
Department of Psychology
University of North Carolina
  at Chapel Hill
reznick@unc.edu

Donna J. Thal, Ph.D.
School of Speech, Language,
  and Hearing Services
San Diego State University
dthal@mail.sdsu.edu

ABOUT THE AUTHORS

Larry Fenson, Ph.D., Professor, Department of Psychology, San Diego State University, 6505 Alvarado Road, Suite 101, San Diego, California 92120

Dr. Fenson received his doctoral degree in child psychology from The University of Iowa. He served as Assistant Professor at the University of Denver and was a National Institute of Child Health and Human Development postdoctoral fellow with Jerome Kagan at Harvard University in Cambridge, Massachusetts. Dr. Fenson has published research on infant attentiveness, early symbolic development, categorization, children's drawing skills, play, and early language assessment. Dr. Fenson chairs the MacArthur-Bates CDI Advisory Board.

Virginia A. Marchman, Ph.D., Research Associate, Department of Psychology, Stanford University, Jordan Hall, Building 420, 450 Serra Mall, Stanford, California 94305

Dr. Marchman holds master of arts and doctoral degrees from the University of California, Berkeley, in developmental psychology and was a postdoctoral fellow at the Center for Research in Language at the University of California, San Diego. She was named Distinguished Scholar at the Callier Center for Communication Disorders and also served on the faculty at the University of Wisconsin–Madison. She is also currently Adjunct Associate Professor in the School of Behavioral and Brain Sciences at The University of Texas at Dallas. She has been on the editorial boards of the *Journal of Speech, Language, and Hearing Research* and *Developmental Psychology*.

Dr. Marchman has conducted research in several areas of language and cognitive development, language disorders, and early childhood development. Her most recent work focuses on the identification of precursors of language delay and individual differences in lexical and morphological development in monolingual English and bilingual (Spanish/English, Chinese/English) speakers. Dr. Marchman is a member of the MacArthur-Bates CDI Advisory Board and is the developer of the CDI Scoring Program.

Donna J. Thal, Ph.D., Distinguished Professor Emeritus, School of Speech, Language, and Hearing Sciences, San Diego State University; Research Scientist, Center for Research in Language, University of California, San Diego, 5500 Campanile Drive, San Diego, California 92182

Dr. Thal holds a master of science degree in speech pathology and audiology from Brooklyn College, New York, and a doctoral degree in speech and hearing sciences from the Graduate School and University Center of the City University of New York (CUNY). She has been a postdoctoral fellow at the Center for Research in Language at the University of California, San Diego (1985–1988), Assistant Professor at Hofstra University in Hempstead, New York (1981–1985), and Assistant Professor at Queens College of CUNY (1979–1981).

Dr. Thal is a developmental psycholinguist and a certified and licensed speech-language pathologist who has conducted research in a number of areas, including typical and disordered development of language and cognition, studies of children with focal brain injury, and studies of children with delayed onset of language. She has also carried out studies of language development in Spanish-speaking infants and toddlers. Her most recent work focuses on early identification of risk for clinically significant language impairment and is funded by an RO1 grant from the National Institute on Deafness and Other Communicative Disorders.

Dr. Thal is an American Speech-Language-Hearing Association (ASHA) fellow. She is also an editorial consultant for language for the *Journal of Speech, Language, and Hearing Research* and the *American Journal of Speech-Language Pathology*. She was the California State nominee for the ASHA Foundation Outstanding Clinical Achievement Award in 1996, received the Monty Distinguished Faculty Award from San Diego State University (SDSU) in 1998, the Albert W. Johnson Research Lecturer Award from SDSU in 1999, and was the Wang Family Excellence Award nominee from SDSU in 2000. She served a 4-year term on the Communicative Disorders Review Committee for the National Institute on Deafness and Other Communicative Disorders (1998–2002). Dr. Thal is a member of the CDI Advisory Board and a co-author of the MacArthur Inventarios del Desarrollo de Habilidades Comunicativas (Paul H. Brookes Publishing Co., 2003).

Philip S. Dale, Ph.D., Professor and Chair, Department of Speech and Hearing Sciences, The University of New Mexico, 1700 Lomas, Albuquerque, New Mexico, 87131

Dr. Dale holds a master of arts degree in communication sciences, a master of science degree in mathematics, and a doctoral degree in communication sciences, all from the University of Michigan, Ann Arbor. He has been Professor of Psychology at the University of Washington, Seattle, and Professor and Chair of Communication Science and Disorders at the University of Missouri–Columbia. His recent research has focused on assessment and interpretation of individual differences in language and literacy development, including behavioral genetic approaches, the relationship of language and literacy, outcomes of early delay, and the effects of early intervention.

Dr. Dale is a Fellow of the American Speech-Language-Hearing Association and of the American Psychological Society. He has served as President of the International Association for the Study of Child Language (1996–1999) and as a member (1993–1997) of the Human Development and Aging-1 Study Section of the National Institutes of Health. He is currently a co-editor of the *Journal of Child Language.* Dr. Dale is a member of the CDI Advisory Board and the primary developer of the MacArthur-Bates Communicative Development Inventory–III (CDI-III).

J. Steven Reznick, Ph.D., Professor, Department of Psychology, University of North Carolina at Chapel Hill, Campus Box #3270, Chapel Hill, North Carolina 27599

Dr. Reznick has held previous appointments at Harvard University in Cambridge, Massachusetts, and Yale University in New Haven, Connecticut. Dr. Reznick's primary research interest is memory development in infants, but his research experience covers a broad range of ages, from birth through adolescence, and topics, including language development, shyness, and autism. Dr. Reznick has been involved with development of the MacArthur-Bates CDIs since their inception, collaborating with Elizabeth Bates on early versions of the instrument and participating in the MacArthur Research Network that supported the formal development of the CDIs. He is a member of the MacArthur-Bates CDI Advisory Board.

Elizabeth Bates, Ph.D., Professor of Cognitive Sciences, University of California at San Diego (In memoriam, 1947–2003)

Elizabeth Bates received her bachelor of arts degree at St. Louis University, Missouri, and earned her doctoral degree in human development from The University of Chicago. She was awarded honorary doctorates from the University of Paris and the New Bulgarian University in Sofia. She was on the faculty of the University of Colorado at Boulder (1974–1981) and was a visiting professor at the University of California, Berkeley (1976–1977). From 1972 until 2003, she was a visiting scholar on a regular basis at the National Research Council Institute of Psychology in Rome. She joined the Psychology Department faculty at the University of California, San Diego (UCSD), in 1982.

Dr. Bates was a founding member of the UCSD Department of Cognitive Science, the first such academic department created in the United States, and served as director of the Center for Research in Language and the Project in Cognitive and Neural Development. She was a co-director of the San Diego State University/UCSD Joint Doctoral Program in Language and Communicative Disorders. Dr. Bates was the driving force behind the MacArthur-Bates CDIs initiatives and a key participant in the MacArthur Research Network that supported their formal development.

ACKNOWLEDGMENTS

We are indebted to many colleagues who assisted us in expanding the geographic and demographic base of our sample. Janna Oetting carried out a special recruitment project that supplied us with a substantial number of primarily African American participants. Terry Cronan, Beverly Goldfield, Letitia Naigles, and Doris Trauner generously contributed CDI data collected in the context of their ongoing research, which supplemented additional data contributed by Virginia Marchman and Donna Thal. Tyler Newton recruited and collected the majority of the CDI: Words and Gestures forms for participants ages 17 and 18 months. Once these data were collected, several people played an invaluable role in turning those CDIs into numbers that could be used in the renorming process. In particular, we thank Suzy Carr Fleisher, Nereyda Hurtado, Elda Jimenez, Carmen Martínez-Sussmann, Maria Martha Moreno, and Laura Smithson for their careful and detail-oriented assistance in data entry, data analysis, and statistical processing of the norming data. Carmen Martínez-Sussmann carried out a literature review on the reliability and validity of the CDIs that was of great assistance in the writing of that section of the manual. We also thank Judith Fenson for her contributions to the development of the expanded CDI scoring guidelines. Finally, we acknowledge the competence and dedication of the professional staff at Paul H. Brookes Publishing Co., including Senior Book Production Editor Nicole Schmidl, Acquisitions Editor Astrid Zuckerman, and former Editorial Director Elaine M. Niefeld.

Because this second edition builds on the work of the first edition, we also acknowledge those who contributed to the original project. We thank the students at the three study sites who worked so hard on the mailings, physical management of the incoming data packets, data scanning and coding, data entry, programming and maintenance of computer records, maintenance of subject records, preparation of tables and figures, handling of inquiries, and execution of the validity studies. In San Diego: Craig April, Hillary Bennett, Dawn Dughi, Robynne Hoffman, Jim McKay, Jennifer Mooney, Michelle Newman, Rosemarie Paris, Mark Polarek, and Tony Ruggieri. In Seattle: Karma Augerot, Amy Julian, Anita Jones, and Cheryl Mercer. In New Haven: Evelyn Backa, Maria Elena Lara, Denise Pinon, Sue Sabatino, Nina Sayer, Wanda Watkins, and Suzanne Zeedyk. Michelle Holt produced all of the final tables and graphs (figures). A special debt is owed to Stewart Burgess, who coordinated the norming project in San Diego.

We also acknowledge the students who contributed to the preliminary norming study in San Diego that provided the empirical basis for the construction of the CDI forms: Sheri Abercrombie, Craig April, Hillary Bennett, Stewart Burgess, Dan Flynn, Jeff Hartung, Michelle Newman, Jordan Omens, Tammy Smith, Vivian Steiner, Susan Robillard, Molly Russell, and Debi Vella.

Technical support was provided by Larry Juarez at the University of California, San Diego, and by Judith Fenson at Children's Hospital, San Diego. We thank our colleagues Donna Jackson-Maldonado and Jerome Sattler for their advice and assistance. Mark Appelbaum and Lee Allard provided us with invaluable guidance in carrying out the curve-fitting procedures.

We would like to express our appreciation to Dr. Joel Snyder in San Diego for his assistance in the recruitment of participants for the normative study and to the Psychology Department Infant Studies Subject Pool Committees at the University of Washington, Seattle, and at the University of California, San Diego, for sharing their mailing lists. Diane Machcinski, Program Manager for the Women, Infants, and Children (WIC) Program administered by the County of San Diego, graciously facilitated our access to participants at several WIC Centers. We were also permitted access to parents at the Hill Health Center in New Haven, Connecticut. In addition, we are grateful to the physicians who assisted in the recruitment of participants in our earlier normative study: Dr. Richard Buchta, Dr. Robert McCord, Dr. Laura Nathanson, Dr. Lisa Stellwagen, and Dr. John Welsh.

This project was funded by the MacArthur Foundation Research Network on Childhood Transitions, chaired by Dr. Robert N. Emde. Matching funds for the purchase of computer equipment were provided by Donald Short, Dean of Sciences, San Diego State University.

*We dedicate this work to Elizabeth Bates.
Research by Liz and her colleagues in the 1970s and 1980s
established the basis for reliable and valid parent report language
inventories. Then, in the late 1980s, Liz became the heart and soul of the
MacArthur Foundation enterprise that led to the creation of the CDIs.
Her energy, enthusiasm and remarkable insight inspired and guided her
MacArthur colleagues in the subsequent expansion of the inventories
and supporting tools. Although Liz's untimely death slowed our
progress, we are confident that her influence is reflected in
this new edition of the manual and that she would be
proud of the success of the enterprise that she
launched and steered so successfully.*

1

INTRODUCTION

OVERVIEW

Parents notice the emergence of language. A child's first words are eagerly awaited, often dutifully recorded in baby books and diaries, and always shared with family and friends. Subsequent progress is noted and enjoyed until the child's language is so far along that it is finally taken for granted. Popular books for parents abound with advice for fostering early communication and guidelines suggesting when language milestones should be reached, but there is no question that early language is salient for parents, and they need no impetus to notice this remarkable aspect of early development. From this perspective, it is surprising that only since the 1980s have parents come to be viewed as a reliable source of information about the young child's communicative skills. The obvious obstacle was to find a technique that allows researchers and clinicians to harvest the parent's rich view of the child's language.

The first systematic attempts to use questionnaires to tap parents' knowledge about their children's language skills were reported by Bates and her colleagues in the 1970s and 1980s (e.g., Bates, Camaioni, & Volterra, 1975). These questionnaires evolved into a set of inventories with detailed questions about vocabulary and grammar. At around the same time, Rescorla (1989) developed a 310-item parent-report checklist of productive vocabulary that was designed as a screening tool for detecting language delay in 2-year-old children. The Mac-Arthur-Bates Communicative Development Inventories (CDIs) build on the foundations laid by each of these earlier initiatives (see section "Origins of the Instruments" in Chapter 4). The first two CDIs (sometimes called *Inventories* in this manual) were published in 1992. These were the CDI: Words and Gestures and the CDI: Words and Sentences. Since that time, the CDIs have been expanded to include one-page brief versions of CDI: Words and Gestures and CDI: Words and Sentences (Fenson, Pethick, et al., 2000). The MacArthur-Bates Communicative Development Inventory–III (CDI-III; described in detail in Chapter 6) was also designed to be used with children from 30 to 37 months of age.

Members of the CDI team have also developed Mexican Spanish versions of CDI: Words and Gestures and CDI: Words and Sentences, as well as brief versions of each of these instruments. The Spanish CDIs and an accompanying manual were published in 2003 (Jackson-Maldonado et al.). In addition, the CDI Advisory Board has authorized and encouraged the adaptation of the CDI forms into a number of other languages. These adaptations are not direct translations to other languages but, rather, assessment tools that take linguistic and cultural differences into account (see Dale, Fenson, & Thal, 1993, & http://www.sci.sdsu.edu/cdi/suggestions_adaptations.htm). A number of these instruments are now available for public use, many with supporting normative data (see the CDI web site, http://www.sci.sdsu.edu/cdi/adaptations.htm, for a complete list of non-English versions of the CDIs). Finally, the CDIs will soon be available in an adaptive-testing format, which uses a computer-based administration of a dynamically selected subset of CDI questions to converge on relevant language parameters quickly and efficiently.

There are two distinct advantages to the strategy of using parents as informants regarding the child's language. First, because the CDIs tap knowledge that most parents and caregivers have about their young children's communicative development, the CDIs lead to a more ecologically valid assessment (Crais, 1995) than commonly used laboratory and clinical measures. Second, the CDI strategy is responsive to Part H of the Education of the Handicapped Act Amendments of 1986 (PL 99-457), Part C of the Individuals with Disabilities Education Act (IDEA) Amendments of 1997 (PL 105-17), and the Individuals with Disabilities Education Improvement Act of 2004 (PL 108-446)—all of which require parent input in child evaluation procedures. Because of these advantages, the CDIs have found wide application among researchers and clinicians.

The clinical utility of the CDIs is particularly noteworthy. Clinicians have found that the CDIs are useful in screening and developing a prognosis for children with language delays (Crais, 1995; Heilmann, Weismer, Evans, & Hollar, 2005; Miller, Sedey, & Miolo, 1995; Thal, Reilly, Seibert, Jeffries, & Fenson, 2004; Yoder, Warren, & McCathren, 1998). Researchers have used the CDIs extensively with a wide variety of populations, including children with language delay, children with Down syndrome and Williams syndrome, bilingual children, children in child care, children from different socioeconomic status (SES) groups, babies who were born preterm or with focal lesions, and so forth (see Chapter 3 for a review of the diverse applications of the CDIs).

This new edition of the manual expands the information presented in the first edition (Fenson et al., 1992/1993) in a number of significant ways:

1. We present an expanded set of normative data that is more demographically balanced than the original norms. The expanded norms also extend the upper age of the CDI: Words and Gestures form to 18 months (formerly 16 months).

2. We provide an overview of the brief versions of the CDIs that parallel the CDI: Words and Gestures form and the CDI: Words and Sentences form.

3. We present detailed information and normative values for the CDI-III, a brief adaptation that is applicable to children 30–37 months of age.

4. More detail is presented on the administration of the Inventories.

5. More detailed directions are provided in the text and appendices on how to tabulate scores for the various sections of the Inventories. Guidelines for scoring the three longest utterances and deriving a mean score (in terms of the mean length of the three longest sentences [M3L]) are greatly expanded, and directions for avoiding common scoring errors are provided.

6. Specific guidelines are provided for using the normative tables for the CDI: Words and Gestures form and the CDI: Words and Sentences form.

7. The section on machine scanning is greatly expanded, and a section is provided on the new option of using desktop scanners.

8. A new CDI automated scoring program is introduced.

9. A new section presents recent data on SES variations in CDI performance and addresses the issue of how scores for various subpopulations should be interpreted.

10. The section on research and clinical applications is updated to reflect new findings.

11. The sections on reliability and validity are greatly expanded, incorporating new data.

One additional change in the CDIs calls for special notice. In December 2003, our beloved colleague Elizabeth Bates died after a long battle with pancreatic cancer. The role that Liz played in the development of the CDIs was vital. The instrument itself was created within Liz's vision of a productive science of child language development, its early stages of development benefited greatly from Liz's nurturance and encouragement, and the continued evolution and impact of the CDIs reflect Liz's influence in every aspect. The CDI team has renamed the Inventories the MacArthur-Bates Communicative Development Inventories to reflect Liz's many contributions.

ORGANIZATION OF THIS MANUAL

The main body of this manual is divided into five chapters. In Chapter 1, methods of assessing early language development are reviewed, the role and value of parent report is considered, and the instruments themselves are described in detail. Chapter 2 provides directions for administering, scoring, and interpreting the CDIs. Chapter 3 outlines possible applications of the CDIs for clinical and research purposes. In Chapter 4, details of the developmental trends for the norming sample are presented, the intercorrelations among the various components of each inventory are described, and measures of the reliability and validity of the instruments are reported. Chapter 5 presents percentile tables and figures for major variables separately for boys and girls and for both sexes combined. Chapter 6 describes the CDI-III.

There are three appendices at the end of the book. Appendix A is the original Basic Information Form that was used in the normative studies to record demographic and other background information about the child and family. Appendix B offers an expanded, photocopiable Basic Information Form that was used in the Spanish normative study and by some of the investigators who contributed data for the expanded CDI norms presented in this book. Appendix C presents the Child Report Forms that provide templates for creating summary sheets for reporting scores. The photocopiable Child Report Forms are useful for research or clinical applications and for distribution to physicians and/or parents when accompanied by an interpretive letter. Versions of these forms are automatically generated by the CDI Scoring Program (see Chapter 2).

METHODS OF ASSESSING EARLY LANGUAGE SKILLS

The language assessment techniques used in research and clinical assessment of infants and toddlers fall into three categories: structured tests, language samples, and parent report. We consider the advantages and disadvantages of each approach.

Structured Tests

In this method, responses are elicited from the child in a relatively formal manner in order to assess the child's knowledge of vocabulary and grammar. Examples of well-known structured tests include the Sequenced Inventory of Communication Development–Revised (SICD-R; Hedrick, Prather, & Tobin, 1984), the Reynell Development Language Scales: U.S. Edition (Reynell & Gruber, 1990), and the Preschool Language Scale, Fourth Edition (PLS-4; Zimmerman, Steiner, & Pond, 2002). Each of these instruments assesses several aspects of communicative development, has been normed on a representative population, and has demonstrated validity and reliability. However, the limitations of structured tests often outweigh their benefits when used with infants and toddlers. Tests require a considerable amount of time to administer, personnel must be trained, and the cooperation of the young child is essential. The latter constraint is particularly problematic for infants and toddlers, who may fear and distrust strangers (e.g., test administrators) and whose cognitive and emotional states vary significantly from hour to hour. The usefulness of structured tests is also limited by their expense, the modest validity that has been demonstrated for most of these instruments when conducted prior to 2½ to 3 years of age, and the inherent problems that arise when standardized tests are used with linguistically and culturally diverse populations (Crais, 1995; Gutierrez-Clellen, 1996; Kayser, 1995; Lahey, 1988; Langdon, 1992b; Mattes & Omark, 1991).

Language Samples

Language sampling is a second popular technique used by researchers and clinicians to gather information about a child's language skills. The aim is to create conditions that prompt the child to talk in a typical manner so that key features of the child's speech can be evaluated. These features include vocabulary range and grammatical complexity. Researchers and clinicians are trained to follow the child's lead, to make conversational responses to the child's utterances, and to ask open-ended questions. Transcription and analysis of naturalistic language samples require highly trained personnel and a substantial amount of time. As a result, most studies incorporating language samples use small numbers of children. Special care needs to be taken when generalizing results from case studies or when data are obtained from a small sample. Another constraint associated with language sampling is that the behavior observed during interactions is highly variable across contexts and interlocutors. In all interactions between a child and another person, it is the dyad that is assessed—whether or not that is the intent of the examiner. Clearly, parent–child interactions differ from those between a child and a specifically trained clinician or researcher. They also differ across parents and across clinicians/researchers, regardless of the level of training. In addition, context has a strong effect on the nature of the behaviors that are observed, especially with young children.

Although a language sample may yield a broader reflection of a child's vocabulary and grammar than a structured test and may provide relatively detailed indices of child language, the method still assesses a restricted range of the child's linguistic abilities. Researchers and clinicians are often most interested in emerging language skills. It is precisely those skills that are unlikely to be observed in a spontaneous play interaction, in which the interlocutor tends to follow the child's lead and purposely refrains from asking pointed or difficult questions.

An additional complication of using language samples emerges from the fact that the technique was developed in the United States with middle-class children who are likely to have had extensive experience with the types of interactions used to obtain the language sample (e.g., Bloom & Lahey, 1978; Lund & Duchan, 1988; Miller, 1981; van Kleeck & Richardson, 1990). These types of interactions may be unfamiliar to children from other cultural groups (Delgado-Gaitán & Trueba, 1991; Farver, 1993; Heath, 1983; Langdon, 1992a; Roopnarine, Johnson, & Hooper, 1994), qualifying the validity of the language samples.

Differences in conversational styles during different types of play interactions are also found within the same cultural or socioeconomic group (Heath, 1983; Laosa, 1982). For example, Jackson-Maldonado (1994) compared the free play language behavior of Spanish-speaking children and parents who were from very low socioeconomic backgrounds in two different play contexts. When provided with a set of colorful plastic toys like those often used in child language research, the mothers typically did not allow their children to play with the colorful toys during the language sampling sessions, saying "Don't touch it" when the children tried to do so. When presented with common household objects found in a local market, such as clay pots, wooden spoons, and fruits or vegetables made from natural materials, however, the mothers eagerly encouraged the children to play with them (Carrillo Aranguren, Jackson-Maldonado, Thal, & Flores, 1997; Jackson-Maldonado, 1997).

Parent Report

The oldest type of parent report is the diary, which has a long and respected history in developmental psycholinguistics (e.g., Dromi, 1987, Hernández-Pina, 1984; Leopold, 1949; Llorach, 1976; López Ornat, Fernandez, Gallo, & Mariscal, 1994; Stern & Stern, 1907; Tomasello, 1992; Truex, 1982). This form of parent report constitutes an invaluable source of information about the child's day-to-day progress in the early stages of language development. However, most diary studies have been published by parent-scientists who have had extensive training in the observation of language behavior—training that the average parent lacks. Nonetheless, the average parent is quite adept at observing his or her child's behavior. Modern-day parent-report instruments have therefore been designed to capture the advantages of the diary study method in a user-friendly format.

Parent report is a component of many widely used screening tools that have been developed for English-speaking infants and toddlers. Examples include the Denver Developmental Screening Test (Frankenburg, Dodds, Fandal, Kazuk, & Cohrs, 1975), the Brigance Inventory of Early Development–Revised (Brigance, 1991), the Birth to Three Developmental Scale (Bangs & Dodson, 1979), the Receptive-Expressive Emergent Language Test, Second Edition (Bzoch & League, 1991), and the Rossetti Infant-Toddler Scale (Rossetti, 1995). Parent report is also incorporated into many structured assessments, such as the SICD-R (Hedric et al., 1984) and the PLS-4 (Zimmerman et al., 2002). Stand-alone parent-report instruments such as the CDIs and the Language Development Scales (Rescorla, 1989) are now widely used with infants and toddlers, both those who speak English and those who speak a variety of the world's languages.

Parent report has a number of inherent advantages over other means of assessing child language. First, because the parent has the opportunity to observe the child in a wide range of situations, parent report can provide data that are more representative of the child's actual language than would be observed in a laboratory sample or a structured test. Second, a child's performance in a laboratory or clinic setting may be strongly influenced by aspects of the child's personality such as shyness and by transient factors such as mood. Parent report should be less susceptible to such factors (Fenson et al., 1992/1993). As Bates, Bretherton, and Snyder (1988) emphasized, parent report reflects "what the child knows," whereas observations at home or in the laboratory are better assessments of "what the child prefers to use" (p. 96). Third, parent report is a cost-effective means for a rapid general evaluation of language that can be valuable for screening purposes in clinical and educational settings as well as research applications. Fourth, parent report can be obtained in advance of actually seeing a child and, therefore, can help in selecting assessment procedures for more in-depth analyses. Clinicians can also use parent report as an adjunct to check the validity of their own evaluations, which would be based on a more limited interaction with the child. Finally, because parent report is based on behavior in contexts outside the clinic or laboratory, it is especially valuable in monitoring changes in language over time—including, when applicable, monitoring the progress of intervention.

Of course, parent report is not without its limitations as a means to assess language abilities (Feldman et al., 2000; Fenson, Bates, et al., 2000; Tomasello & Mervis, 1994). Parents may be accused of being biased observers, tending to either under- or overestimate their child's developing abilities, but other domains of development appear to be more vulnerable to this bias than is language. For example, Reznick and Schwartz (2001) asked mothers to rate their child's tendency to behave intentionally (using a parent-report questionnaire) and to rate their child's language development (using a CDI). One group of mothers made these ratings longitudinally when infants were 8, 10, and 12 months old, and three other groups of mothers made ratings cross-sectionally when their infants were at comparable ages. Successive ratings of intentionality were higher in the longitudinal cohort, suggesting that mothers altered their view of the infant (or their behavior toward the infant) due to the assessment experience. In contrast, CDI scores were identical for mothers completing them repeatedly or for the first time. This finding suggests that language assessment may be relatively objective. Moreover, the assessment context per se can be altered to enhance the objectivity of assessment. For example, Fenson and colleagues argued that parent report is most likely to be accurate under two conditions: 1) when assessment is limited to current and emergent behaviors and 2) when a recognition format is used. Each of these conditions places fewer demands on the respondent's memory, relative to retrospective and/or free-form reports. The recognition strategy capitalizes on the greater ease of picking out possible examples from a set, as contrasted with recalling those examples anew. The perspective underlying the CDIs is that it is better to ask parents to report on their child's vocabulary by selecting words from a comprehensive or representative list rather than to have them write down all of the words they can recall hearing their child use. The recognition format also reduces the need for parents to make inferences about the nature of the questions being asked and/or their child's level of ability relative to other children (e.g., "What do they mean by animal words?" "What do they mean by 'lots' of animal words?").

DESCRIPTION OF THE INVENTORIES

The CDIs are designed to be completed by parents, to profit from the advantages of good parent diaries, and to minimize the limitations of language samples and structured tests. Specifically, the CDIs target current and emerging behaviors, rely on recognition memory for specific information, and avoid retrospective accounts. The CDIs are easy to administer and interpret and allow researchers to collect comparable data on a small scale or a large scale. The general effectiveness of the CDIs, specifically their reliability and validity in the assessment of key language milestones, is documented in detail in the sections in Chapter 4 called "Reliability of the Inventories" and "Validity of the Inventories."

The goal of the CDIs is to yield reliable information on the course of language development from children's early signs of comprehension, to their first nonverbal gestural signals, to the expansion of early vocabulary and the beginnings of grammar. Because language changes so dramatically during the period from 8 to 30 months, it was necessary to develop two separate forms designed for different age ranges.

The CDI: Words and Gestures form, appropriate for use with 8- to 18-month-old typically developing children, generates scores for vocabulary comprehension, vocabulary production, and the use of communicative and symbolic gestures. Users who are familiar with the first edition of the CDIs will note that the upper age limit for CDI: Words and Gestures has been extended by 2 months in this second edition. The upper age limit was extended because few ceiling effects were observed at 16 months on key variables in the normative study and many clinicians and researchers are interested in obtaining information about receptive vocabulary and gesture use in children up to 18 months of age. In some cases, it may be appropriate to use CDI: Words and Gestures with children who are chronologically older than 18 months. (See the section called "Evaluation of Older Children with Language Delay" in Chapter 3 for information about the use of CDI: Words and Gestures with older children who may have delays in language development.)

The CDI: Words and Sentences form, designed for 16- to 30-month olds, yields scores for vocabulary production and a number of aspects of grammatical development, including sentence complexity and the mean length of the child's longest utterances. Because word comprehension usually grows so rapidly during the second year of life, it is unrealistic to expect parents to accurately appraise their child's vocabulary and distinguish between the words their child says and the words their child knows much beyond the middle of the second year. Hence, the vocabulary section of the CDI: Words and Sentences form is limited to expressive language. The second edition of CDI: Words and Sentences covers an age range identical to that in the first edition.

The norms for forms of the CDI permit a child's scores on the major components of each inventory to be converted to percentile scores, reflecting the child's rank relative in comparison with other children of the same age and sex. The following two sections provide more specific information on each of the two forms.

CDI: Words and Gestures

The CDI: Words and Gestures form comprises two major parts (see Table 1.1). Part I, Early Words, begins with three short subsections. Section A, First Signs of Understanding, includes three questions designed to determine whether the child has begun to respond to language at all. In Section B, Phrases, the parent chooses the phrases that the child understands from a 28-item list. Section C, Starting to Talk, includes two questions, one asking parents about the frequency with which the child imitates words or phrases and one about the frequency with which the child labels objects.

The major portion of Part I is a 396-item Vocabulary Checklist. Here, parents indicate which words their child understands and which words their child understands and says. The CDI: Words and Gestures form targets both vocabulary comprehension and production in the 8- to 18-month age range because in-

Table 1.1. Description of the components of the CDI: Words and Gestures form

Part I: Early Words

A.	First Signs of Understanding	General questions about early comprehension of familiar words and phrases (3 items), designed to determine if the child has begun to respond to language
B.	Phrases	Comprehension of everyday phrases and routines (28 items)
C.	Starting to Talk	Imitation and labeling (2 items)
D.	Vocabulary Checklist	A 396-item checklist organized into 19 semantic categories, with separate columns for comprehension (understands) and production (understands and says)

Part II: Actions and Gestures

A.	First Communicative Gestures	
B.	Games and Routines	A through E (63 items) form the Total Gestures summary score.
C.	Actions with Objects	A through B (18 items) form the Early Gestures summary score.
D.	Pretending to Be a Parent	C through E (45 items) form the Later Gestures summary score.
E.	Imitating Other Adult Actions	

formation about comprehension vocabulary is particularly important during the months when spoken language is still minimal. In addition, longitudinal studies of infants and toddlers have suggested that language comprehension is a better predictor of later language development (Bates et al., 1988) and of persistent language impairment than is language production during the early stages of development (for a review, see Thal & Katich, 1996). A category of production without understanding was not included because we discovered in extensive pilot work that most parents assume that a word produced is also a word understood.

The Vocabulary Checklist is organized into 19 semantic categories. Ten of the categories contain nouns (Animal Names, Vehicles, Toys, Food and Drink, Clothing, Body Parts, Furniture and Rooms, Small Household Items, Outside Things and Places to Go, and People). Additional sections include words in the following categories: Sound Effects and Animal Sounds, Games and Routines, Action Words (verbs), Words about Time, Descriptive Words (adjectives), Pronouns, Question Words, Prepositions and Locations, and Quantifiers and Adverbs.

Part II of the CDI: Words and Gestures form focuses on the child's use of communicative and symbolic actions/gestures. This section offers an opportunity for appraisal of a range of early communicative and representational skills that are not dependent on verbal expression. Gestures have been shown to play an important role in an infant's early developing communicative skills (Bates, Benigni, Bretherton, Camaioni, & Volterra, 1979; Caselli, 1990). Research has also revealed that gestures may serve as an index of early symbolic skill and as a cornerstone of linguistic development (Acredolo & Goodwyn, 1985, 1988; Bates et al., 1979; Bates et al., 1988; Butterworth & Morrisette, 1996; Capirci, Iverson, Pizzuto, & Volterra, 1996; Goldin-Meadow & Morford, 1985; Iverson, Capirci, & Caselli, 1994; Pérez & Castro, 1988; Piaget, 1962; Thal & Bates, 1988; Thal & Tobias, 1992, 1994; Thal, Tobias, & Morrison, 1991). Part II complements the linguistic items indexed in Part I and may be especially useful for assessing communicative and symbolic skills in infants who have little expressive language and in children who are demonstrating signs of language delay or impairment (Terrell & Schwartz, 1988; Terrell, Schwartz, Prelock, & Messick 1984; Thal & Tobias, 1992, 1994; Thal et al., 1991).

The 63 gestures are organized into five categories. The items in Section A, First Communicative Gestures, signal the onset of intentional communication, an important prerequisite for language. These include the deictic gestures of giving, showing, pointing, and reaching, as well as a number of conventionalized communicative gestures (e.g., shaking the head "no"). Often, these early gestures are combined with vocalizations in making requests or in drawing an adult's attention to something (e.g., Bates et al., 1979; Rollins & Snow, 1998). The items in Section B, Games and Routines, form an important part of the early social interactive basis for communicative development (Bruner, 1977). The most common items in Sections A and B typically are seen in a majority of children well before the end of the first year of life (Bates et al., 1975; Bates et al., 1979; Locke 1978). Results from a number of studies of preverbal development suggest that the gestures in Section A are strongly predictive of the emergence of meaningful speech (Bates et al., 1979; Thal & Bates, 1989). For example, many children nod or shake their head before they use the words "yes" and "no" or reach for an object to request it before they use the object's name to request it. The predictive value of the gestures in Section B is less well known, although there is evidence that children's participation in social games and routines has a key role to play in the regulation and maintenance of joint attention (Rollins & Snow, 1998; Tomasello & Ferrar, 1986). Taken together, the items in Sections A and B compose the Early Gestures summary score.

The child's use of gestures such as those in Section C, Actions with Objects, and Section E, Imitating Other Adult Actions, expresses a growing understanding of the world of objects and the uses of things (Bretherton, 1984; Piaget, 1952). The child's appropriate use of objects distinguishes these actions from the earlier undifferentiated responses of the younger infant and signals an emerging representational capacity (Fenson, Kagan, Kearsley, & Zelazo, 1976). The earliest of these schemes begins to appear in children's play well before the end of the first year. Others appear late in the first year and early in the second year (McCune-Nicolich & Fenson, 1984). The items in Section D, Pretending to Be a Parent, are among the first types of true symbolic gestures, preceded only by similar actions directed toward the self (Piaget, 1962). These types of actions generally emerge a few months later in the child's spontaneous play than the accommodative acts in Sections C and E (Fenson & Ramsay, 1980). The sum of responses in Sections C, D, and E forms the Later Gestures summary score.

CDI: Words and Sentences

The CDI: Words and Sentences form is designed for use with children between 16 and 30 months of age and assesses various aspects of the acquisition of vocabulary and grammar. Table 1.2 provides an overview of the sections of the CDI: Words and Sentences form.

The general format for the CDI: Words and Sentences form is similar to that of the CDI: Words and Gestures form; however, there are several age-related

Table 1.2. Description of the components of the CDI: Words and Sentences form

Part I: Words Children Use	
A. Vocabulary Checklist	Classification of whether the child says words in 22 semantic categories (680 items)
B. How Children Use Words	Use of language to refer to the past, the future, and absent objects and people (5 items)
Part II: Sentences and Grammar	
A. Word Endings/Part 1	Questions about the child's use of language to refer to the past, the future, and absent objects and people (4 items)
B. Word Forms	A list of irregular plural nouns (5 items) and irregular past tense verbs (20 items)
C. Word Endings/Part 2	A list of overregularized nouns (14 items) and overregularized verbs (31 items)
Combining	A question about whether the child has begun to combine words (1 item)
D. Examples	A request to write examples of the three longest sentences that the parent has heard the child say in the recent past (basis for the mean length of the three longest sentences [M3L])
E. Complexity	Sentence pairs that contrast in length and grammatical complexity (37 item pairs); asks the parent to indicate which one sounds most like the way the child currently talks

differences (see Table 1.2). Part I, Words Children Use, contains a 680-word vo-cabulary checklist. In contrast to the CDI: Words and Gestures form, the Vo-cabulary Checklist on the CDI: Words and Sentences form is limited to language production, asking parents to only indicate the words that their child says. This is due to our discovery in successive phases of pilot testing that parents are less likely to be able to keep track of both comprehension and production as their child's expressive language begins to grow rapidly toward the end of the second year of life. The CDI: Words and Sentences form has a greater number of words than the CDI: Words and Gestures form because of expected age-related increases in vocabulary.

The Vocabulary Checklist is organized into 22 semantic categories. In gen-eral, these categories directly parallel those included on the vocabulary check-list on the CDI: Words and Gestures form. Eleven of these categories contain only nouns (Animals, Vehicles [Real or Toy], Toys, Food and Drink, Clothing, Body Parts, Small Household Items, Furniture and Rooms, Outside Things, Places to Go, and People). Additional categories include Sound Effects and Animal Sounds, Games and Routines, Action Words, Descriptive Words, Words about Time, Pronouns, Question Words, Prepositions and Locations, Quantifiers and Articles, Helping Verbs, and Connecting Words. On the CDI: Words and Sen-tences form, Outside Things (#10) and Places to Go (#11) appear as separate cate-gories. Articles are combined with Quantifiers in a single category (#20).

During the period from 16 to 30 months of age, language use is also char-acterized by word combinations, emerging syntax, and increasingly complex use of morphological forms. In order to capture this developmental information, Part II of the CDI: Words and Sentences form, Sentences and Grammar, focuses on the assessment of several aspects of morphology and syntax. The first three sections assess production of selected regular and irregular bound morphemes. Section A, Word Endings/Part 1, contains 4 questions that address the child's use of the regular plural (-s), possessives (-'s), progressive (-ing), and past tense (-ed). Section B, Word Forms, asks parents to specify whether the child has begun to use each of 5 common irregular plural nouns and 20 common irregular past tense verbs. Section C, Word Endings/Part 2, is a checklist of 14 commonly overregularized plural nouns (e.g., "teeths," "blockses") and 31 overregularized past tense verb forms (e.g., "blowed," "sitted").

The latter portion of Part II focuses on multiword utterances. Following Section C, parents are asked whether the child has begun to produce word combinations. If parents select *Not Yet*, they are instructed to stop at that point and not complete the subsequent sections, D and E.

In Section D, Examples, parents are asked to provide examples of their child's most complex early utterances—that is, to write down examples of the three longest utterances that they have heard their child say recently. This method is based on the work of Rescorla (1989) and has been used in versions of the CDIs in other languages. These example sentences yield an index of morphosyntax that is strongly correlated with mean length of utterance (MLU) from spontaneous language samples in English (Dale, 1991) and in Spanish (Thal, Jackson-Maldonado, & Acosta, 2000). (See the section in Chapter 4 called "Validity of the Inventories" for more information). It is included so that clinicians and researchers can have an additional index of toddler speech that is based on the child's actual utterances. M3L is calculated by computing the average number of morphemes in the example sentences provided by the parent (i.e., counting the number of morphemes in the three examples and dividing by 3).

In Section E, Complexity, parents are asked to choose which member of each of 37 phrase/sentence pairs best reflects the way their child talks. In each case, the second member of each pair is the more advanced form. To provide an adequate developmental range, the items were selected to evaluate production of bound morphemes (Items 1–12), function words (Items 13–24), and early-emerging complex sentences (Items 25–37).

Guidelines for Choosing Between the CDI: Words and Gestures and the CDI: Words and Sentences Forms in the 16- to 18-Month Age Range

In the 16- to 18-month range, CDI users have the option of choosing either the CDI: Words and Gestures form or the CDI: Words and Sentences form. Selection of one form over the other depends on the specific aims of the investigator. Here are some considerations to aid in making the best choice.

FOR ASSESSMENT THAT WILL NOT CONTINUE PAST 18 MONTHS
Reasons for Choosing CDI: Words and Gestures

- If interested in gestures and/or vocabulary comprehension

- If interested in comparing children's scores on vocabulary comprehension and production

- If interested in comparing children's scores on vocabulary comprehension and production with gesture scores

- If interested in tracking a child's scores on one or more measures across the 8- to 18-month age range

Reasons for Choosing CDI: Words and Sentences

- If interested in obtaining measures of early grammatical skill
- If there is reason to expect relatively large vocabularies, and therefore a need for a longer word list, or there is specific interest in a subset of vocabulary that has limited representation in CDI: Words and Gestures

Note: The grammatical skills measured by the CDIs are often at a beginning or preemergent stage in the 16- to 18-month period. Thus, the CDI: Words and Gestures form may offer a richer picture of communicative development in this range because most children develop comprehension vocabulary and gestures by the 16- to 18-month period.

FOR ASSESSMENT THAT BEGINS AT OR BEFORE 18 MONTHS AND CONTINUES BEYOND THAT AGE IN EITHER CROSS-SECTIONAL OR LONGITUDINAL SAMPLES

Reasons for Choosing CDI: Words and Gestures (at or younger than 18 months)

- If interested in comparing a child's standing on vocabulary comprehension and/or gestures with grammatical skills beyond 18 months
- If there is reason to expect language development is proceeding more slowly than the typical rate of development

Reasons for Choosing CDI: Words and Sentences

- If interested in cross-sectional or longitudinal comparisons on the same scales when testing begins in the 16- to 18-month age range and when it continues beyond 18 months

THE MACARTHUR-BATES COMMUNICATIVE DEVELOPMENT INVENTORY SHORT FORMS

Despite the efficiency and statistical integrity of the CDIs, the time needed to complete the form and the requirement that the parents be literate restrict the applicability of the CDIs in some research, clinical, and educational settings when a rapid assessment of a child's language level is needed. The short forms were developed to capitalize on the demonstrated effectiveness of parent input in a briefer format. These forms can be completed in less than 10 minutes and, when necessary, can be administered by interview to parents with limited or absent literacy skills (although normative data using an interactive approach has not been collected). The CDI short forms provide reliable indices of vocabulary development that are highly correlated with vocabulary scores on the full CDIs.

Separate forms are available for 8- to 16-month-old children (Level 1) and for 16- to 30-month-olds (Level 2). The Level 1 version contains an 89-word vocabulary checklist with separate columns for comprehension and production. There are two equivalent Level 2 forms. Either can be used for a single administration. In addition, a question appears at the bottom of each of these two forms, asking parents if their child has begun to combine words, with the 3 response options being *not yet, sometimes,* and *often.*

These forms should be of value to researchers and clinicians who are seeking a quick assessment of early language. The forms may be particularly valuable when time and/or parental literacy is limited. The short forms may also prove useful in longitudinal studies, in which repeated administration of the full inventory may be impractical. For children in the 16- to 30-month age range, investigators have the option of alternating between the two equivalent forms to reduce effects accruing from repeated administration of the same items. The forms may also be useful for children with developmental delays who are beyond the specified age ranges for typically developing children.

Because the short forms include only vocabulary measures, and a much briefer list than in the full forms, they are not likely to be as precise as the full CDI. For example, the word list is too brief to be useful for studies of vocabulary composition (Bates et al., 1994). Also, the brevity of the list exacerbates the ceiling effect after 27–28 months, especially for children with higher abilities. Finally, the Level 2 forms do not include any measure of grammatical development following the emergence of word combinations. Researchers and clinicians should carefully consider their goals in language assessment prior to selecting a particular form. Detailed information about the CDI short forms and normative data can be found in Fenson, Pethick, et al. (2000).

2

ADMINISTRATION, SCORING, AND INTERPRETATION

ADMINISTERING THE INVENTORIES

It takes approximately 20–40 minutes to complete a CDI form, depending on the extent of the child's communicative skills. The administration of the Inventories and the Basic Information Form is designed to be self-explanatory. Nevertheless, researchers and clinicians (and relevant staff) who plan to use the Inventories are strongly encouraged to become thoroughly familiar with the guidelines for their administration in order to provide timely and accurate answers for any questions that emerge. We provide an overview of general administration issues in this section.

General Instructions

Written instructions are provided at the beginning of each section of the Inventories. In the original normative study, parents received and returned the form by mail. An accompanying letter explained the scientific purpose of the project, but the only directions about filling out the form were those that appeared on the form itself. For most parents, these instructions are all that will be necessary.

On occasion, parents may have questions about various aspects of the process. For those parents, and any others who could potentially need additional guidance, the examiner may wish to read and explain the instructions aloud and/or provide an additional handout that gives an overview of important points. The expanded norms described in the present edition combine the data from the original study with newly collected data in which additional reminders and instructions may have been used. Thus, the norms are based on a mixture of instructional contexts. We see this variability in instructions as enhancing the generalizability of the norms. It is useful to remind parents about all of the following items:

- Indicate **Today's date** and **Child's birth date** on form.

  Parents should be shown where to indicate these dates, as they are crucial in the calculation of the age of the child at the time of administration. It is often useful to double-check the birth year because parents often mistakenly put the current year instead.

- Complete the **Basic Information Form** (Appendix B).

  To provide background information, Appendix A presents a limited version of the Basic Information Form, which was used in the original CDI normative study. Appendix B provides an expanded, photocopiable version of this form, and this is the questionnaire that should be used for obtaining basic contact, demographic, and medical history information.

- Please **read instructions** carefully!

  The written instructions can be highlighted directly on the form and/or shown to the parents. When necessary, instructions may be read (or summarized) for the parent, and the procedures for completing specific sections may be further elaborated verbally. It is helpful to highlight the Vocabulary Checklist and to elaborate on the difference between the replies *Understands* and *Understands and Says*.

- Do not mark **imitations.**

  It is of utmost importance that parents realize that they should not probe for production by testing the child's ability to imitate a word or gesture. Rather, they should mark only words the child uses spontaneously, without a direct model. If possible, parents should fill out the questionnaire during a quiet time away from the child (e.g., during naptime) so that they will not be distracted and, more important, will not be tempted to probe or confirm hypotheses about what the child says and understands.

- Give the child credit for **mispronounced or "baby talk" words** (e.g., saying "nana" instead of "banana" or "banky" instead of "blanket").

  Parents should be reminded that children sometimes have their own special words for things or people. These words are acceptable substitutes for items listed on the Vocabulary Checklist.

- Give the child credit for **words the child says or understands that have the same meaning** as a word on the CDI.

  A child may use or understand different words that have the same meaning of words on Vocabulary Checklist. These words may be particular to the family or the child or to where the family currently resides.

- Take into account **words indicating the names of people** (e.g., *Tati* or *Oma* instead of *Grandma*) or words **that are specific to your dialect/region** (e.g., *owie* instead of *booboo*, *sack* instead of *bag*, *pop* instead of *soda*).

  If the forms are to be scored by hand and additional information is wanted, parents should be told to check the word on the CDI form and to write the word that the child uses next to the word on the form. If the forms are to be scored by machine, it is important to avoid stray marks that may lead to scanner errors; thus, parents should be told to check the word on the form that means the same thing as the word the child produces but not to write in the word itself.

- **Ask others** (e.g., nanny, child care providers, other family members) to help you fill out this form.

    In some cases, parents may only have access to a portion of the situations in which children's language abilities are demonstrated—for example, when children are attending a child care program. It may be appropriate to have multiple individuals complete the forms (e.g., mothers and grandmothers). In instances where children are exposed to more than one language, it is important that the person most familiar with the child's competence in English complete the appropriate English CDI form. Input can be sought from others familiar with the child's understanding or use of English. Input should not be sought from informants about the child's competencies in other languages when completing the forms in English. On page 38, we discuss recommended procedures for assessing the linguistic competencies of children who are receiving exposure to more than one language. We suggest that parents note the names of all individuals who completed the forms on the front cover of the Inventory. We believe that the advantage of using multiple informants is that it provides the most representative sample of what the child knows. Marchman and Martínez-Sussmann (2002) compared the use of both strategies to use of single informants by correlating the results with spontaneous language samples. They found that having multiple informants increased the validity for some variables and never decreased the validity, providing support for this strategy. However, the norms are based on a single informant methodology, and that must be kept in mind if multiple informants are used.

- Make sure you **complete all pages of the form.**

    Parents may be less likely to skip pages if they are shown the entire form ahead of time. It is often useful to page through the completed form to make sure that all pages have been completed.

- Please use a **No. 2 pencil** to fill in the bubbles.

    A No. 2 pencil is required if the forms are to be scanned by an Optical Mark Reading (OMR) machine that is not capable of detecting marks made with ink. (For more information about machine scoring, see the section in this chapter called "Automating the Scoring Process.")

Other Administration Considerations

Parents who have low literacy levels may have difficulty or feel apprehensive about reading and completing the forms. If this is the case, it may be best for examiners to fill out the form with the parents. Although some users report that they have assisted parents by telephone, no data are available on the possible effects of this strategy.

An additional concern arises when the English-language CDIs are used in conjunction with CDIs in other languages with bilingual children (e.g., in assessments of children who are learning both English and Spanish). In these cases, it is particularly important to query the parents regarding their proficiency in either or both languages prior to their completion of the forms. In some cases, a single parent may not have the language skill to complete both

Inventories. For example, in a bilingual household in which the mother primarily speaks English but the father primarily speaks Spanish, it would not be appropriate for the mother to complete both an English CDI and a Spanish CDI. Again, we suggest that parents indicate who completed each form on the cover.

Finally, it is strongly recommended that the Inventories be checked immediately upon receipt for completeness and potential inconsistencies across sections. For example, a parent may indicate that the child combines words sometimes or often but then does not provide example sentences. Follow-up contacts may be necessary to fill in missing portions of the Inventories. Furthermore, it may be necessary to probe for accuracy if the information provided on the form is strikingly disparate with age-based expectations (e.g., a 30-month-old with only 10 words produced; a 12-month-old with 300 words produced). Probes should be as neutral and nonthreatening as possible and should seek to clarify whether the parent understood the instructions. For example, the examiner might ask the parent, "I see that you reported that Johnny can say 'now.' Can you give me an example of a situation in which he might say that word?" The parent may then volunteer that Johnny says that word "whenever I ask him to say it or whenever he hears me say it." This would indicate that the parent was inappropriately marking words that the child only produces in imitation but does not necessarily understand or use spontaneously.

SCORING AND INTERPRETING THE INVENTORIES

Users of the Inventories have several scoring options and computerized tools at their disposal. The Inventories are easily scored by hand, with percentile scores computed by comparing raw totals with the values in the look-up tables. Tables 2.1 and 2.2 give pertinent information for scoring and interpreting the CDI: Words and Gestures form and CDI: Words and Sentences form, respectively. The Child Report Forms provide a convenient format to present summary scores (totals) and percentile values that can be given to the parent (see Appendix C and the subsections in this chapter called "Using the Norms" and "Obtaining and Interpreting Children's Scores"). These are also useful summary records for researchers, clinicians, physicians or other professionals.

Hand scoring of the Inventories is most convenient for small numbers of forms when the objective is to obtain summary scores for the various sections of the inventories. Scoring the inventory by hand, including looking up percentiles and completing the Child Report Form, typically requires 20–30 minutes, depending on the child's age and language skill.

Alternatively, users may select from a variety of tools that automate the process of tabulating and summarizing the data on the Inventories. Computer-based tools for use with the Inventories have become more cost-effective and user-friendly since the late 1990s. For example, programs such as the CDI Scoring Program (http://www.sci.sdsu.edu/cdi/scoringdb_p.htm) interface with data that are hand entered or read by scanner, automatically tabulate summary scores, generate Child Report Forms, and track client information in a database.

Table 2.1.   Scoring the CDI: Words and Gestures form

Section of CDI	How to score
Part I: Early Words	
A. First Signs of Understanding	For each item, record *yes* or *no* responses.
B. Phrases	Count and record the number of *understands* responses across all items.
C. Starting to Talk	For both items, record *sometimes* and *often* responses as *yes*. Record *never* responses as *no*.
D. Vocabulary Checklist	Words Produced: Obtain the score for vocabulary production by adding the number of *understands and says* responses marked by the parent across each of the 19 categories (396 maximum).
	Words Understood: Obtain the total score for vocabulary comprehension by adding the number of items across all 19 categories for which the parent marked either *understands* OR *understands and says*. Blanks are not counted. If the parent marked both response alternatives for an item, treat it as if the parent has marked only the *understands and says* column (as it is inclusive). Note that the score for vocabulary production will never exceed but can equal the score for vocabulary comprehension. However, the score for vocabulary comprehension will almost always exceed the score for production.
Part II: Actions and Gestures	
A. First Communicative Gestures	Count *sometimes* and *often* responses as *yes* (12 items total). If both are marked, include the item in the count. Treat blank responses as *not yet*.
B. Games and Routines	
C. Actions with Objects	Count the number of *yes* responses in each section (51 items total). Treat blank responses as *no*.
D. Pretending to Be a Parent	
E. Imitating Other Adult Actions	

To compute summary scores:
- *Total Gestures:* Sum and record the number of *yes* responses in Sections A through E (63 maximum).
- *Early Gestures:* Sum and record the number of *yes* responses in Sections A and B (18 maximum).
- *Later Gestures:* Sum and record the number of *yes* responses in Sections C through E (45 maximum).

Regardless of the specific method chosen, we suggest that all users familiarize themselves with the general process and logic of scoring the Inventories. We provide step-by-step instructions on scoring in Tables 2.1 (CDI: Words and Gestures) and 2.2 (CDI: Words and Sentences).

Scoring Examples

In general, scoring involves counting responses, summing scores, looking up normative values, and completing the summary sheet. Additional scoring guidelines and examples are provided in this subsection for selected measures. For clarity, the examples are further grouped by form type (i.e., CDI: Words and Gestures or CDI: Words and Sentences).

Examples from the CDI: Words and Gestures Form

Example of Obtaining a Vocabulary Score   Across all categories in the Vocabulary Checklist section of Part I (Early Words) of the CDI: Words and Gestures form, sum the number of items in the *understands* and *understands and says* columns. The Total Comprehension score is the sum of both columns. The Total Production score is the sum of only the *understands and says* col-

Table 2.2. Scoring the CDI: Words and Sentences form

Section of CDI	How to score
Part I: Words Children Use	
A. Vocabulary Checklist	Count the number of responses in each subsection. Do not count items left blank. *To compute a summary score:* • Words Produced: Sum and record the number of *says* (i.e., selected) responses across all 22 categories (680 maximum).
B. How Children Use Words	For each of the 5 items, record *sometimes* and *often* responses as *yes*. Record *not yet* responses as *no*. Count items left blank as *no*.
Part II: Sentences and Grammar	
A. Word Endings/Part 1	For each of the 4 items (which concern regular suffixes), record *sometimes* and *often* responses as *yes*. Record *not yet* responses as *no*. Count items left blank as *no*.
B. Word Forms	For the 5 irregular nouns and 20 irregular verbs, count the number of *yes* (i.e., selected) responses in each section. Count items left blank as *no*.
C. Word Endings/Part 2	For the 14 overregularized nouns and 31 overregularized verbs, count the number of selected responses across the Noun and Verb sections to obtain a single total score.
Combining	Record *sometimes* and *often* responses as *yes*. Record *not yet* as *no*. If the item is left blank, count the response as *no*.
D. Examples	Count and record the number of morphemes in each example utterance (maximum of 3) provided by the parent. *To compute a summary score:* • Mean length of the three longest sentences (M3L): Sum the number of morphemes in each example; divide by 3. If fewer than three examples are provided, divide by the number provided (1 or 2). If *not yet* is marked for combining, score M3L as 1. • The process of obtaining the M3L score requires more than just simple counts of marked items. Detailed instructions on how to score the three longest utterances and obtain the M3L are provided in the "Scoring the Child's Three Longest Sentences" section of Chapter 2.
E. Complexity	Count and record the number of items in which the *second* (more complex) of the two alternatives (37 maximum) is marked. If both alternatives are chosen, score as if the parent chose only the second. Do not count items left blank. If *not yet* is marked for combining, score Complexity as 0.

umn. The most common error in scoring vocabulary for the CDI: Words and Gestures occurs when counting total number of words for Total Comprehension. If the parent marked the *understands and says* column for a word, that item contributes to the totals for both Total Comprehension and Total Production scores. If only the *understands* column is marked, that item contributes to the Total Comprehension score but *not* the Total Production score. If the parent marked both *understands* and *understands and says*, treat it as if the parent only marked *understands and says*. Note that the score for Total Production will never exceed the score for Total Comprehension, but the score for Total Comprehension will generally exceed the score for Total Production. In the following example, looking only at the Vehicles (Real or Toy) subsection of the CDI: Words and Gestures Vocabulary Checklist, the child would be credited for understanding 4 words and producing 2 words.

3. VEHICLES (Real or Toy) (9)								
	under-stands	under-stands and says		under-stands	under-stands and says		under-stands	under-stands and says
airplane	●	○	car	○	●	stroller	●	○
bicycle	○	○	firetruck	○	○	train	●	●
bus	○	○	motorcycle	○	○	truck	○	○

Examples of Obtaining Gesture Scores   In Part II (Actions and Gestures), Section A (First Communicative Gestures), credit the child with the gesture if either *sometimes* or *often* is marked. Blanks are not counted at all. In the following example, the total number of gestures used by the child is 6.

A. FIRST COMMUNICATIVE GESTURES			
When infants are first learning to communicate, they often use gestures to make their wishes known. For each item below, mark the line that describes your child's actions right now.	Not Yet	Sometimes	Often
1. Extends arm to show you something he/she is holding.	○	●	○
2. Reaches out and gives you a toy or some object that he/she is holding.	○	●	●
3. Points (with arm and index finger extended) at some interesting object or event.	○	○	●
4. Waves bye-bye on his/her own when someone leaves.	○	●	○
5. Extends his/her arm upward to signal a wish to be picked up.	○	●	○
6. Shakes head "no".	○	○	○
7. Nods head "yes".	●	○	○
8. Gestures "hush" by placing finger to lips.	●	○	○
9. Requests something by extending arm and opening and closing hand.	○	●	○
10. Blows kisses from a distance.	○	○	○
11. Smacks lips in a "yum yum" gesture to indicate that something taste good.	○	○	○
12. Shrugs to indicate "all gone" or "where'd it go".	○	○	○

For the remaining 4 categories in the Actions and Gestures section, credit the child with the gesture only if the *yes* column is marked. Blanks are counted as *no*. In the following example, the child is credited with 3 gestures. Refer to Table 2.1 for summing scores across the sections into scores for Total Gestures, Early Gestures, and Later Gestures.

B. GAMES AND ROUTINES		
Does your child do any of the following?	Yes	No
1. Play peekaboo.	●	○
2. Play patty cake.	●	○
3. Play "so big".	○	●
4. Play chasing games.	●	○
5. Sing.	○	○
6. Dance.	○	●

Examples from the CDI: Words and Sentences Form

Example of Obtaining a Production Score   Across all of the sections on the Vocabulary Checklist in Part I (Words Children Use) of the CDI: Words and Sentences form, credit the child with the word if it is marked. Blanks are not counted at all. In the following example, which shows only the Sound Effects and Animal Sounds and Animals (Real or Toy) sections, the total number of words produced by the child is 10.

1. SOUND EFFECTS AND ANIMAL SOUNDS (12)					
baa baa	●	meow	●	uh oh	○
choo choo	●	moo	●	vroom	●
cockadoodledoo	○	ouch	○	woof woof	●
grrr	○	quack quack	●	yum yum	○

2. ANIMALS (Real or Toy) (43)					
alligator	○	duck	●	penguin	○
animal	○	elephant	○	pig	○
ant	○	fish	○	pony	○
bear	○	frog	○	puppy	○
bee	○	giraffe	○	rooster	○
bird	○	goose	○	sheep	○
bug	○	hen	○	squirrel	○
bunny	○	horse	○	teddybear	○
butterfly	○	kitty	○	tiger	○
cat	●	lamb	○	turkey	○
chicken	○	lion	○	turtle	○
cow	○	monkey	○	wolf	○
deer	○	moose	○	zebra	○
dog	●	mouse	○		
donkey	○	owl	○		

Scoring the Child's Three Longest Sentences   Section D (Examples) is scored by determining the number of morphemes per sentence. Scoring of this section is more complex than other sections of the inventory. Morpheme coding should only be done by individuals who are familiar with the guidelines for marking morphemes in child English as set forth in Brown (1973) and Miller (1981). First, we provide some general guidelines for coding morphemes. Then, we provide a number of specific examples of the types of phrases common in young children's speech.

If the parent marked *not yet* in response to the Combining question, mean length of the three longest sentences (M3L) should be scored as 1. If fewer than three examples are provided, compute M3L based on the number of examples available (one or two). If an example consists of more than one sentence, it should be broken into its component sentences. If this procedure results in more than three total sentences, the three longest resultant sentences in the complete set of examples should be used to compute M3L.

Sentences consisting of more than one independent clause that are not connected by a conjunction such as *and* but are separated by a comma, colon, or semi-colon (indicating separation of ideas) should be counted as separate sentences. For example, "I belong here, I'm a smart boy" should be counted as two sentences. An exception is if the independent clauses appear to be contrastive and are of a parallel structure; in this case, the example should be counted as 1 utterance—for example, "You take this one, I'll take that one."

Sentences with one or more instances of the word *and* or *then* should be counted as 1 utterance. For example, "I want to get out and put on a dress and go downstairs and play."

Sentences that are clearly routines—such as songs, nursery rhymes, and poems—should be excluded. Examples include "Happy birthday to you," "The wheels of the bus go 'round and 'round," "Humpty Dumpty sat on a wall," and "I love you, you love me." Note: "I love you" is counted as a sentence if it is not part of a response that is a routine.

Use the following guidelines to determine the number of morphemes. Examples are provided for reference.

Determining number of morphemes:

The number of morphemes per sentence is determined in general accordance with the guidelines summarized in Miller (1981). In some cases, words should be divided into morphemes that are counted separately. In other cases, words or common phrases are counted as a single morpheme. In the examples that follow, the critical items are indicated in bold.

1. *The following are counted as separate morphemes:*

Regular inflectional suffixes (third person singular, past, progressive, plural, possessive, and plural possessive)

Child says	Morpheme breakdown	Total morphemes
He **goes**	he **go es**	3 morphemes
I **opened** the door	I **open ed** the door	5 morphemes
Her is **crying**	her is **cry ing**	4 morphemes
Want big **shoes**	want big **shoe s**	4 morphemes
Mommy's car	**Mommy s** car	3 morphemes

Contractions:

Child says	Morpheme breakdown	Total morphemes
I **don't** want to go	I **do n't** want to go	6 morphemes
He's my little brother	**he s** my little brother	5 morphemes

Overregularizations:

Child says	Morpheme breakdown	Total morphemes
He **falled** down	he **fall ed** down	4 morphemes

2. *The following are counted as one morpheme:*

Irregular forms and diminutives:

Child says	Morpheme breakdown	Total morphemes
He **went** outside	he **went** outside	3 morphemes
Horsie has big **teeth**	**horsie** has big **teeth**	4 morphemes

Semi-auxiliaries/catenatives (e.g., "wanna," "gonna"):

Child says	Morpheme breakdown	Total morphemes
I **wanna** eat dinner	I **wanna** eat dinner	4 morphemes

Compound words, proper nouns, and "frozen phrases":

Child says	Morpheme breakdown	Total morphemes
I want **orange juice**	I want **orangejuice**	3 morphemes
Burger King is my favorite	**BurgerKing** is my favorite	4 morphemes
drink **all gone**	drink **allgone**	2 morphemes

Note: Fillers such as "um," "uh," "ah," and "oh" are not counted as morphemes. However, exclamations that introduce sentences (e.g., "oh," "hey") should be counted as morphemes.

Scoring Complexity   The grammatical Complexity score is derived by summing the number of times the parent chose the second of the two examples. Blanks are not counted. If the child is not reported to be combining words, the child's complexity score should be 0. In the following example (showing just the first section of Part II, Section E), the child would be credited with a complexity score of 4.

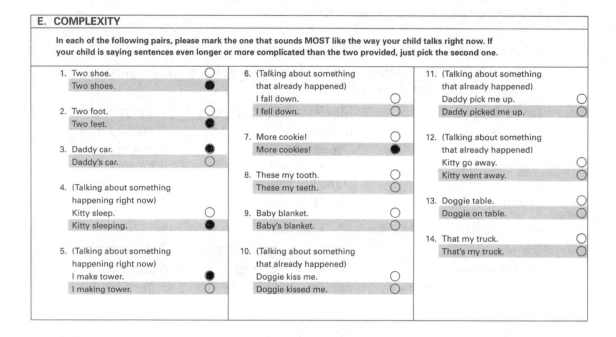

Automating the Scoring Process

Tools are available that automate some or all of the scoring process. Use of these tools can reduce the time required to score the Inventories and increase the accuracy. In this section, we first review the process of machine-scanning the Inventories and then describe tools that are available to automate the scoring process—in particular, the CDI Scoring Program. Users who plan to do all scoring by hand, can skip ahead to the section called "Using the Norms." It should be noted, however, that the CDI Scoring Program does not require machine-scanned data; users may hand count the Inventories and still automate the processes of computing summary scores, looking up percentiles, and generating reports. Thus, the section called "CDI Scoring Program" may be relevant even to users who are not scanning completed Inventories.

Machine Scanning   Only original forms (not photocopies or forms created for image scanners) can be used for machine scanning. This process involves some type of Optical Mark Reading (OMR) system. All OMR systems require a scanner connected to a computer and a software program that is compatible with the scanner. These systems automatically read the completed Inventory form and create a data file in ASCII format, which is essentially a single, long row of 1s and 0s for each scanned inventory. The scanned data output can then be converted to meaningful Inventory categories (e.g., total number of words produced) with the use of a program designed for or adapted to that purpose (e.g., the CDI Scoring program). Examiners may supplement the Inventory forms with a user-completed "header sheet" that allows additional information to be added to each child's scanned record (e.g., child's birth date, test date). Any additional information of this type may also be entered by keyboard, depending on the particular scanning software being used. For the CDI: Words and Sentences form, the M3L must be calculated by hand and then may be added to the header sheet or by keyboard.

As of 2006, two types of OMR systems are available. First, a traditional OMR reader (e.g., National Computer Systems [NCS], Scantron)—the kind that is commonly associated with standardized testing, preprinted forms, and No. 2 pencils—can be used. Some newer types of OMR scanners can read forms completed in ink or pencil. Second, forms can be scanned using an image scanner, a device that is becoming an increasingly common accompaniment to personal computers. Both types of automated scoring systems require a modest to substantial investment in hardware and software, as well as an initial programming of software. In the CDI norming study, the forms were scanned into a PC-compatible computer using a NCS scanner and the NCS ScanTools software. OMR scanners also require periodic maintenance (e.g., recalibration).

Traditional OMR scanners generally involve an investment of at least several thousand dollars or more. These systems are designed specifically for the purpose of scanning large numbers of standardized forms and incorporate features intended to maximize scanning speed and accuracy. For example, these systems have the capacity to process thousands of forms per hour, to automatically feed forms into the scanner, and to simultaneously read the front and back of the page in a single pass (using a "dual-read heads" feature). In our experience, traditional OMR systems are generally quite accurate and can process a completed Inventory in less than 30 seconds. Traditional OMR scanners accept forms that are filled out with No. 2 pencils. Users should take care to become familiar with the requirements of their particular scanner before purchasing inventory forms.

Desktop image scanners are generally a less expensive option (starting at less than $100 but ranging as high as $3,000) for the machine scoring of the Inventories. However, these systems are considerably slower and typically require more page handling by the user (e.g., turning over the pages). The forms can be completed using a pen or any type of pencil. More expensive image scanners will give the user faster scanning rates (although still not as fast as traditional OMR readers), and they often come with accessories that reduce the amount of form handling by the user (e.g., an automatic form feeder). Using this type of system, an average of 2–3 minutes per form is required to complete the scanning process.

As mentioned previously, both systems require software (e.g., ScanTools, Remark) that converts the OMR information to a data file. Most traditional OMR scanners bundle the form-reading software when the hardware is purchased. Because desktop image scanners are used for a variety of other purposes (e.g., scanning photographs), the software necessary for reading the Inventories is generally not sold along with the scanner hardware. However, several form-reading software products are compatible with a wide range of image scanners. We are most familiar with Remark Office OMR by Principia Products, although users may wish to explore other alternatives before making a final selection.

For both traditional and desktop scanning systems, the setup of the OMR software involves configuring the program to read the format of the Inventories (i.e., where the bubbles are and in what order to put them in the output file). Once the scanning system has been set up, processing the forms is a clerical task, although technical advice is likely to be necessary from time to time for hardware and software problems. See the CDI web page for template configurations that were used to process the Inventories for the norming studies (http://www.sci.sdsu.edu/cdi/scoring_t.htm). There are two types of templates: one for use with NCS ScanTools software for traditional OMR readers and the other for use with Remark Office by Principia Products for desktop scanners.

As noted, there are various choices in scanning technology. Users should take care to order the forms that match their scanning hardware and/or software.

CDI Scoring Program   The CDI Scoring program is designed to facilitate the tabulation, percentile calculation, report generation, and data-tracking functions associated with the use of the English and Spanish forms. The CDI Scoring Program is not available for Mac platforms, but it runs on PCs equipped with Microsoft Windows 95, 98, or XP and Microsoft Office 97, 2000, or XP (with Microsoft Access, Word, and Excel). (For more information, see http://www.sci.sdsu.edu/cdi/scoringdb_p.htm.) Versions are available that process all of the CDI forms, including the English CDIs (CDI: Words and Gestures and CDI: Words and Sentences) and the Spanish CDIs (Inventarios I and II), as well as the brief forms in English (Levels I, IIA, and IIB) and in Spanish (I, II).

Data from the Inventories can be incorporated into the CDI Scoring Program in two ways. Users who hand score the Inventories can input data into the program by keyboard. On-screen windows allow data entry at either the category level (e.g., Sound Effects and Animal Sounds) or the item level (e.g., quack quack). Users who choose the machine-scanning option can import scanner output that is generated by either traditional or image scanner systems directly into the CDI Scoring Program. The scanner output must have a fixed column starting point, and each scanned form should be in a single file. Other constraints about how the scanner output data are interpreted by the program are specified more fully at http://www.sci.sdsu.edu/cdi/scoringdb_p.htm.

The CDI Scoring Program automates several aspects of the scoring process and provides additional data tracking and analyses tools. Specifically, the program does the following:

- It automatically calculates percentiles for key variables that are included in reports to parents or for in-house use. The program can also calculate composite vocabulary scores that reflect responses from both the English CDIs and the Spanish Inventories (Pearson, Fernandez, & Oller, 1993, 1993/1995;

Umbel, Pearson, Fernandez, & Oller, 1992). This feature is appropriate when English and Spanish Inventories are available for a given child at or near the same age (see also Marchman & Martínez-Sussmann, 2002).

- The program automatically generates Child Report Forms in both English and Spanish. The program also generates a cover letter that is intended to accompany the Child Report Form. Letter templates can be modified to meet the users' own specific needs and can be tailored for several subpopulations (e.g., a set for typically developing children, a set for children with delayed language development). See the CDI web site for examples of Child Report Forms and parent letters for both the English and Spanish Inventories (http://www.sci.sdsu.edu/cdi/scoringdb_p.htm).

- The program provides database management and tracking tools by storing data from the CDIs, as well as a variety of demographic and medical information, as provided on the Basic Information Form (see Appendix B).

- The program generates summaries of data, selecting participants by any criterion and outputting any variable from the Inventories and/or user-defined variables. These can be output into a table (in Microsoft Access format) or spreadsheet (in Microsoft Excel format), which can then be imported to statistical packages as needed.

Choosing a Scoring Option   Three factors should be considered when making a decision about which procedures to adopt for scoring the Inventories: 1) the number of forms to be processed; 2) the level of data description and analyses of interest; and 3) the availability of support personnel for programming and maintaining computers and scanners.

Number of Forms to Be Processed   Given the necessary equipment and technical support or the possibility of outside scanning arrangements, machine scanning is the best option for users who plan relatively large-scale, long-term endeavors. The decision to use machine scanning should also be made in the context of the types of data that are to be analyzed. Given the wide range of potential uses of the Inventories, it is difficult to specify a precise number of forms at which scanning would become more expedient than hand scoring, although 150–200 is a good estimate. If the number of forms to be processed does not warrant the investment of machine scanning, hand scorers may still use the CDI Scoring Program to automate the computation of summary scores and percentiles, and the generation of Child Report Forms.

Level of Data Description and Analyses of Interest   Scanning is a particularly attractive option when the user is interested in analyses at the individual item level as well as at the category level. The alternative to scanning when individual item data are of interest is to enter each data point by keyboard into a computer file. Entering individual item data requires 883 data points per child for the CDI: Words and Gestures form (28 values for comprehension of phrases, 396 values for word comprehension [understands], 396 values for word production [understands and says], 63 values for gestures and actions), plus additional columns for designating the child's subject number, birth date, and so forth. The CDI: Words and Sentences form requires more than 700 data points. Inputting the data is a labor-intensive endeavor, even with a modest number of forms, and some data entry errors must be expected. Of course, a clinician or researcher interested in examining item data for an individual child would not need to scan forms for this purpose. A child's knowledge of specific words or types of words could be easily evaluated by hand tabulation. Here, data entry templates have prespecified slots for each item, reducing possible confusion across items. Furthermore, the program imports default values into the templates so that only items that differ from that default value need to be entered by the user via the keyboard (i.e., *no* is the default response, so only *yes* responses need to be entered). Use of the CDI Scoring Program significantly reduces the time required and the potential for errors.

Availability of Support Personnel Machine scanning requires hardware and software that many researchers and clinicians do not have readily available; thus, they must invest in the hardware and software if they are interested in machine scanning. However, some schools, hospitals, and universities already have the equipment necessary for scanning forms using this method and, when provided with the appropriate software templates, users may be able to scan inventories on a contract basis. The availability of these resources may significantly reduce the start-up costs associated with machine scanning using traditional OMR systems. As mentioned previously, desktop scanners are becoming increasingly available in many university and clinical settings. The conversion of these desktop scanners to process CDI forms may require the purchase and configuration of software.

Once a machine scanning system is in place, the scanning of the forms becomes a clerical task. It should be kept in mind that prior to scanning, a few minutes of preparation time are generally required for each form in order to perform various operations that ensure the integrity of the data. These include checking that each response bubble is appropriately filled in, penciling over responses marked in ink when traditional scanners are being used, erasing stray marks, making sure that no pages have been inadvertently skipped, separating the pages for insertion into the scanner, copying the subject number onto each page (in case the stack of forms should be dropped), and preparing the header sheets. The preparation time may equal that required for hand scoring. Nonetheless, when the individual item data are of interest, users may want to consider machine scanning.

Using the Norms

The percentile scores provided in Chapter 5 allow establishment of the status of individual children relative to their age-mates on each major section of CDI: Words and Gestures and CDI: Words and Sentences forms. For example, Table 5.5 shows the percentile scores associated with vocabulary comprehension (Words Understood) totals for girls for each month on the CDI: Words and Gestures form. A 12-month-old girl reported as understanding 90 words would have a percentile score of 55 (i.e., just above the middle of the distribution for that month). A girl of the same age with a score of 216 would fall at the 90th percentile, placing her in the top 10% of her age group. Of course, children's raw scores will usually not precisely match the values listed in the percentile tables. For guidelines on how to determine percentile scores for raw scores that fall between two tabled values, see the section "More Specific Guidelines for Computing Percentiles." The Child Report Forms for the CDI: Words and Gestures and the CDI: Words and Sentences forms, which appear in Appendix C, provide a convenient format to summarize the scores and percentiles for a given child.

As in the first edition of the CDI manual, the tabled values are "smoothed" scores, which were derived by plotting the best-fitting linear or logistic curve through the raw percentile scores (in 5 percentile increments: 5th, 10th, 15th, and so forth) for each inventory summary score. This procedure compensates for irregularities in raw scores produced by random variation. These data are presented in graphic form in Chapter 5 (Figures 5.1 through 5.33).

For most measures on both the CDI: Words and Gestures form and the CDI: Words and Sentences form, mean scores tend to be higher for females than for males of the same age. As a consequence, females often reach various milestones (e.g., age at which 50% of the sample are reported to exhibit a given behavior) 1–2 months earlier than males. Although the magnitude of the differences between the two sexes is usually quite small and the differences are statistically reliable at only a few of the monthly intervals, sex differences are often of interest in evaluating the pace of development of individual children; hence, for most measures, separate tables are provided for the two sexes.

For most research and clinical purposes, it is recommended that percentile scores be computed on the basis of both age and sex. For the convenience of users who wish to score forms without reference to sex, however, fitted percentile tables for the sexes combined are also presented for each major scale (see Tables 5.1, 5.4, 5.7, 5.10, 5.13, 5.16, 5.19, 5.22, 5.25, 5.28, and 5.31). For all of the percentile tables, children should be assigned the highest rank that applies. For example, in Table 5.8, a 9-month-old girl with a raw score of 2 should be assigned a percentile score of 60. In Table 5.9, a 10-month-old boy with a raw score of 4 should be assigned a percentile score of 75.

Percentile scores are not appropriate for some sections of each form (e.g., the How Children Use Words and Combining sections of the CDI: Words and Sentences form). Tables are provided that show the percent of children reported to use the specific linguistic form (e.g., Tables 4.20 and 4.24 in Chapter 4) for each of those sections.

In all cases, caution should be exercised when applying the norms to children from families in which the parents have very low education and/or socioeconomic levels, and to children whose chronological ages exceed the upper limits of the inventories. (See the section in this chapter called "Using the Norms with Children from Families of Low Socioeconomic Status" and the section in Chapter 3 called "Evaluation of Older Children with Language Delay.")

Obtaining and Interpreting Children's Scores

This section covers methods for obtaining and interpreting scores on the CDI: Words and Gestures form and the CDI: Words and Sentences form, as well as more specific guidelines for computing percentiles and additional considerations. In addition, coverage is given to the special topics of using the norms with children from families of low socioeconomic status and with children who are learning more than one language.

CDI: Words and Gestures   Three major features of communicative development can be derived from the CDI: Words and Gestures form: comprehension of words and phrases (from the Vocabulary Checklist), production of words (from the Vocabulary Checklist), and production of actions and gestures (from Part II: Actions and Gestures). The CDI: Words and Gestures form also includes two other sections (First Signs of Understanding and Starting to Talk) that do not provide percentile scores. Table 2.3 provides specific instructions for interpreting scores from the CDI: Words and Gestures form.

CDI: Words and Sentences   Eight sections, five of which yield percentile scores, are provided by the CDI: Words and Sentences form. The five that yield percentile scores are the Vocabulary Checklist, Word Forms, Word Endings/Part 2, Examples (M3L), and Complexity. In developing profiles for individual children, the examiner can also make use of scores on How Children Use Words, Word Endings/Part 1, and Combining by consulting the percent distri-

Table 2.3.   Interpreting scores from the CDI: Words and Gestures form

Section of CDI	Descriptive statistics/ developmental trends	Percentile tables	Directions for evaluating a child's scores
Part I: Early Words			
A. First Signs of Understanding	Table 4.6	N/A	Note that 78.1% of the 8-month-old girls and 75.0% of the 8-month-old boys were reported to be exhibiting each of these 3 items. By 11 months, nearly all of the children were reported to be exhibiting all 3 items.
B. Phrases	Figures 4.1 and 4.2 Tables 4.7 and 4.8	Tables 5.1 5.2, and 5.3	Use the percentile tables for Phrases Understood (28 items).
C. Starting to Talk	Figure 4.3 Table 4.9	N/A	For each of these 2 items, compare the child's status with the percent of age-mates for whom parents gave affirmative (*sometimes* or *often*) responses.
D. Vocabulary Checklist	Figures 4.4 through 4.7 Tables 4.10 through 4.13	Tables 5.4 through 5.9	Use the percentile tables for Words Understood and Words Produced, counted separately (396 maximum each).
Part II: Actions and Gestures			
A through E: Total Gestures	Figures 4.8 and 4.9 Tables 4.14 and 4.15	Tables 5.10, 5.11, and 5.12	Use the percentile tables for Total Gestures (Sections A though E: 64 items), or use the tables for Early Gestures (Sections A and B: 18 items) and Later Gestures (Sections C through E: 45 items) computed separately.
A and B: Early Gestures	Table 4.16	Tables 5.13, 5.14, and 5.15	
C through E: Later Gestures	Table 4.16	Tables 5.16., 5.17, and 5.18	In most cases, Total Gestures is the most appropriate score, but depending on the age/developmental level of a particular child, users may find that breaking scores into Early Gestures and Later Gestures provides more detailed information about a given child's status.

bution tables. Table 2.4 provides specific instructions for interpreting the data on the CDI: Words and Sentences form.

Percentile rank tables provide a convenient method for identifying where an individual child falls within a group. Percentile values can be derived from the look-up tables (see Chapter 5) or generated automatically with the CDI Scoring Program. Here we outline the general instructions for determining percentile ranks and percent distributions. These instructions are particularly useful when percentile equivalences are scored and derived by hand; however, we recommend that all users familiarize themselves with the logic of the process, even if automated procedures are applied.

The steps that allow the determination of percentile scores are as follows:

1. Determine responses or Summary Scores using the guidelines in Table 2.1 (for CDI: Words and Gestures) or Table 2.2 (for CDI: Words and Sentences).

2. Find the table that corresponds to the subscale for the child's gender. For example, use Table 5.5 for Words Understood for girls on the CDI: Words and Gestures form, and use Table 5.21 for Words Produced for boys on the CDI: Words and Sentences form.

3. Select the column for the child's age and find the number closest to the child's raw score. (See "More Specific Guidelines for Computing Percentiles" for information on situations in which the raw score falls between two numbers.)

4. Align this number with the column on the far left to obtain the percentile equivalence.

5. If the raw score corresponds to two or more percentiles, select the highest one that applies.

More Specific Guidelines for Computing Percentiles If the child's score corresponds exactly to a number in the table, assign that exact percentile equivalence score. For example, using Table 5.5, a 13-month-old girl who is reported to comprehend 53 words falls at the 20th percentile. In other words, 20% of the 13-month-old girls in the norming sample had a vocabulary comprehension score that was at or below 53 words. A 14-month-old girl reported to understand 141 words would have a 50th percentile score (i.e., the score falls at the middle of the distribution for that month). A girl of the same age with a score of 280 words would fall at the 90th percentile, placing her in the top 10% of her age group.

If the child's score falls between two numbers in the table, there are two ways to assign a percentile value. It is reasonable to use the conservative strategy of giving the percentile that is below the real score. For example, if a 13-month-old girl was reported to comprehend 59 words, that score would fall between the 20th (53 words) and the 25th (63 words) percentiles. Conservatively, she would be placed at the 20th percentile. The most accurate method, however, is to interpolate between percentiles and assign an exact percentile. The tabled values of 53 and 63 would differ by 10 words. The child's score is 6 points above the lower value of 53 and is therefore $^{6}/_{10}$ of the way between the two tabled values. The entire interval corresponds to a 5-percentile difference (between the 20th and

Table 2.4.   Interpreting scores from the CDI: Words and Sentences form

Section of CDI	Descriptive statistics/ developmental trends	Percentiles	Directions for evaluating a child's scores
Part I: Words Children Use			
A. Vocabulary Checklist	Figures 4.10 and 4.11 Tables 4.17 and 4.18	Tables 5.19, 5.20, and 5.21	Use the percentile tables for Words Produced (680 maximum).
B. How Children Use Words	Figures 4.12 and 4.13 Tables 4.19 and 4.20	N/A	Table 4.19 allows the user to compare the child's pace of acquisition of these four terms, which refer to temporal and special displacement. Compare the sum with the mean and median number of affirmative responses (*sometimes* plus *often*) at that child's age. On the basis of this table, a child's ability can be scored as average, above average, or below average for age in the use of each of these concepts.
Part II: Sentences and Grammar			
A. Word Endings/Part 1	Figure 4.14 Table 4.21	N/A	Table 4.21 summarizes the normative scores for these 4 word forms. Compare the child's status—*not yet, sometimes,* or *often,* with *sometimes* or *often* indicating an affirmative response—with the percentage of agemates reported to be using each form. As in Part IB, the child's performance can be compared with that of other children to make a judgment concerning the child's pace of acquisition of these features of language.
B. Word Forms	Figure 4.15 Table 4.22	Tables 5.22, 5.23, and 5.24	Use percentile table for Word Forms. Infrequent use of irregular nouns and verbs by most children prior to 23 or 24 months produces poor discrimination between adjacent percentile levels up to that age and at even older ages for low-scoring children. For example, at as late as 22 or 23 months, the addition of a single item can produce a jump of 15 or 20 percentile points. Hence, the percentile scores for children younger than 24 months should be interpreted very cautiously and are best regarded as a rough approximation of the child's relative pace of development for this measure. As the reported use of irregular endings increases, the percentile rankings become less sensitive to minor variations in raw scores.
C. Word Endings/Part 2	Table 4.23 Figure 4.16	Tables 5.25, 5.26, and 5.27	Table 4.23 allows the user to compare the child's pace of acquisition of overregularized words with that of other children of the same age. Because of the slow emergence of overregularized words during the first half of the third year, this measure will not be effective in distinguishing children who are slow to demonstrate these errors from children who fall closer to the mean. The children who stand out on this measure will be those reported to use a large number of these forms. That is, the measure may be more sensitive to acceleration in the use of these forms than to delay. We do not have sufficient information to know whether frequent and early use of these terms is a reliable indicator of a broader acceleration in the pace of language acquisition.

(continued)

Table 2.4. *continued*

Section of CDI	Descriptive statistics/ developmental trends	Percentiles	Directions for evaluating a child's scores
Combining	Figure 4.17 Table 4.24	N/A	Table 4.24 shows the percentage of girls and boys at each monthly interval reported to be combining words (i.e., those for whom parents gave either *sometimes* or *often* responses).
D. Examples	Figures 4.18 and 4.19 Table 4.25	Tables 5.28, 5.29, and 5.30	Use percentile tables for mean length of the three longest sentences (M3L). For children whose parents gave a *not yet* response or *no* response in the Combining section, assign an M3L of 1.0. See Table 2.2 and the Chapter 2 instructions ("Scoring the Child's Three Longest Sentences") for more information.
E. Complexity	Figures 4.20 and 4.21 Tables 4.26 and 4.27	Tables 5.31, 5.32, and 5.33	For children who are combining words, the Complexity section provides a relative index of the grammatical sophistication of the child's utterances. Use percentile tables for Complexity (37 maximum). Due to the considerable range of variability in typically developing children, the margin of error should be regarded as relatively wide at all ages. Small differences in percentile rankings between individual children or between groups of children should be interpreted with caution. In addition, a substantial number of girls younger than 22 months and boys younger than 23 months are not yet combining words and therefore score 0. Consequently, the measure is of limited value for general evaluation of grammar at those ages.

25th percentiles)—$\frac{6}{10}$ ($\frac{3}{5}$) of that 5-percentile difference yields a value of 3; adding the value of 3 to the 20th percentile assigns the child a percentile score of 23.

For sections in which percentile tables are not available, use the tables that present the distributions of children by age in order to estimate how the child's score compares with that of age-mates. For example, Table 4.24 shows the percentage of children at each age with affirmative responses on Combining (Note: In such cases, affirmative responses represent the sum of *sometimes* and *often* responses). A 28-month-old boy whose parent reports that he is not combining words would fall in the lowest 4.7% of 28-month-old boys in the norming sample. Table 4.20 shows the distribution of How Children Use Words. A 21-month-old child whose parent reports that he or she does not talk about absent objects would fall in the lowest 18.9% of children at this age, as 81.1% of 21-month-old children are reported to refer to absent objects. If the parent reports that the same child talks about events that occurred in the past, the child would be placed in the upper 56.8% of the children in the norming sample of the same age.

Additional Considerations   In evaluating percentile scores, it is important to examine the distribution of the raw scores at that age. For ages at which the skills in question are just emerging, scores are compressed, so very small differences in raw scores can sometimes produce large shifts in percentile scores.

As seen in Table 5.9 in Chapter 5, for example, for 8-month-old boys, the entire range in scores for Words Produced is 10. For this same measure, an 11-month-old boy not yet credited with any words would be assigned a percentile score of 35. A child of the same age credited with 9 words would be placed 45 percentile points higher at 80%. At older ages, a difference of 9 words can result in a gain of only 1 or 2 percentile points. Vocabulary production presents the most extreme instances of score compression, but there are several other measures for which a restricted range in raw scores when a skill is just emerging creates unstable percentile levels (e.g., Complexity—see Tables 5.31, 5.32, and 5.33). Because relatively few items can have such a large effect on the child's percentile scores in these instances, users should be very cautious in drawing strong conclusions based on these reported values.

Using the Norms with Children from Families of Low Socioeconomic Status
Although the original normative sample was relatively large, it was principally middle to upper middle class in composition, thus underrepresenting the lower education and lower socioeconomic segments of the U.S. population. In this second edition, the composition of the sample is improved in at least three ways. First, the proportion of non-white participants is now 26.9% compared with 13.1% in the original sample (Fenson et al., 1992/1993). Second, more families are included in which mothers have completed 12 years of education or less (31.5% compared with 22.4%). Finally, the data set has been expanded geographically, sampling children who are living in Midwestern states (Wisconsin) and Southern states (Texas, Louisiana), as well as on the East and West coasts (New Haven, Seattle, San Diego). As presented in Chapter 4, however, the current normative sample still does not fully reflect the U.S. population in terms of educational level or ethnicity. Thus, although the second edition includes considerable improvements, users of the Inventories should be aware of the character of the norming sample and should be cautious when using the norms with children and families from low educational and/or socioeconomic levels. Some examples of demographic variation in the prior sample and the current sample are provided next.

The analyses reported in Chapter 4 revealed several SES-related effects: For the CDI: Words and Gestures form, there were higher mean scores for Phrases Understood, Vocabulary Comprehension, and Total Gestures among 8- to 12-month-old children of mothers whose education terminated with high school. The SES results for the CDI: Words and Sentences form also paralleled the findings of the original data set, with better scores credited to the higher SES groups on the main measures.

A normative study of the Mexican Spanish MacArthur-Bates Communicative Development Inventories (Jackson-Maldonado et al., 2003) found the same inverse relation between mother's educational level and infant vocabulary comprehension. The Mexican sample was more demographically balanced than the English sample, permitting a fuller analysis of SES effects. Three maternal education levels were compared: no high school, some high school, and some college. Mean vocabulary comprehension scores for mothers who had the least education were significantly higher than those of children with the most education. As in the English data, this finding was limited to the 8- to 12-month old group, with no SES differences found in the 13- to 16-month-old group. The more familiar positive relation between SES and language skills was found for the three main CDI: Words and Sentences scales (Words Produced, Examples/ M3L, and Complexity). For each scale, this effect was limited to the oldest of the three age groups (26–30 months).

Feldman et al. (2000) reported additional data on the influence of socio-economic variables on CDI scores. They tested more than 2,000 children longitudinally, once when they were between 10 and 13 months of age and another time when the children were between 22 and 25 months of age. Paralleling both the English and Spanish normative studies, Feldman and colleagues found that mean scores for two CDI: Words and Gestures measures (Words Understood and Words Produced) were highest for children of mothers without a high school education, intermediate for children of high school graduates, and lowest for children of college graduates. For another CDI: Words and Gestures measure (Words Understood), the scores of children with less than high school and high school graduates were equivalent, but both were higher than scores for children of college graduates. A pattern of increasing scores with decreasing education also applied in the Feldman et al. data for one CDI: Words and Sentences measure (Word Endings/Part 2). However, two other CDI: Words and Sentences measures (Examples/M3L and Complexity) showed the more familiar positive relation between SES and language skills.

Taken together, these studies suggest that some mothers with lower educational levels overestimate or at least overreport their children's comprehension vocabularies during the earliest phase of vocabulary development between 8 and 13 months of age. The Feldman et al. (2000) data indicate that some mothers with very low education might also overestimate or overreport certain newly emerging language skills in toddlers as well. However, the total amount of variance accounted for by SES was quite small in all three studies. In the original English norming study, the variance accounted for by SES was less than 2% for all of the CDI: Words and Gestures and CDI: Words and Sentences measures. A similar degree of variance accounted was found in the second edition as well (see Chapter 4). In the Spanish norms, the variance accounted for by each of the CDI: Words and Gestures measures was less than 2%; for the CDI: Words and Sentences measures, the values were less than 2% for Words Produced and 2% for Examples/M3L and for Complexity. In the Feldman study, SES accounted for 3.8%–7.1% of the variance in the CDI: Words and Gestures sample and 1.6%– 5.1% in the CDI: Words and Sentences sample. The higher variance scores in the Spanish and Feldman samples would be expected, given their greater demographic breadth relative to the English samples.

Note that overreporting and/or overestimating was most likely to occur in both the English and Spanish norming studies for scales that require inference. In the study by Feldman and colleagues (2000), it also occurred for phrases understood and for vocabulary production. Although vocabulary production would certainly seem to require less inference than judgments about the comprehension of words or phrases, Feldman et al. pointed out that production at 1 year of age also requires some degree of inference (due to the lower intelligibility of speech at this age for some children). The measures for which Feldman et al. obtained negative correlations with measures of SES (Word Forms and

Word Endings/Part 2) also require more inference than do the CDI: Words and Sentences measures for which a positive relation was obtained between language level and SES.

Are the CDIs Valid for Children from Families with Low Socioeconomic Status?
Further evidence for negative effects of socioeconomic factors on CDI toddler scores was found by Arriaga, Fenson, Cronan, and Pethick (1998). These investigators evaluated scores on CDI: Words and Sentences forms completed by the mothers of 103 children who had older siblings participating in Head Start programs. By definition, these were low-income parents. A matching sample of 103 toddlers from middle-income families was drawn from the English norming study. The scores for the children from the Head Start families were substantially lower for the Words Produced and for the two grammatical measures (the Combining and Complexity sections). For all three scales, the distribution of scores for the children from low-income families was displaced approximately 30% toward the lower end of the middle-income distribution. For example, the Words Produced scores for 82.5% of the low-income sample fell below the median scores contained in this manual. Similar results were obtained for the Complexity scale (78.5%).

Arriaga et al. (1998) identified two possible sources of the lower CDI scores reported for children from families with low SES. An environmental deficiency hypothesis asserts that these children acquire language skills at a slower rate than middle-class children as a consequence of a less favorable language environment. This hypothesis implies that the lower scores received by children from families with low SES are authentic. Note that probable inflation in the percentile tables means that the scores of these children would have been perhaps not quite as low as their tabled values had the norming sample been more demographically balanced (specifically, if the sample had been less skewed toward middle-income families.)

A second hypothesis—parent misjudgment—attributes lower scores to parents underreporting on the CDI forms, implying that children's language skills are better than their CDI scores reflect. If this effect is widespread, it would result in significant underestimation of the language skills of children from low-income families. Underreporting by parents with low SES would not necessarily preclude the use of the CDIs for this segment of the population. The CDIs should provide a general idea of a child's language skills relative to other children of the same age. Underreporting would, however, result in the assignment of percentile scores that are below the child's true ability level. Percentile scores obtained on children from low-income families should therefore be interpreted with extra caution.

None of the studies reviewed allow a determination of whether the lower scores reflected underreporting by parents, deficient skills in the children, or some combination of these factors. Roberts, Burchinal, and Durham (1999) used an abbreviated, preliminary version of the CDI: Words and Sentences short form in a study that revealed evidence for a significant amount of underreporting by some parents with low SES. In a sample of 87 low-income families, CDI scores were lower than data obtained from direct testing and observational measures.

Yet, this effect was found only at 30 months and did not occur at 18 or 24 months. There are, moreover, a number of limitations to the Roberts et al. study. First, comparisons were made between the CDI: Words and Sentences Words Produced scores and scores on the Expressive subscale of the Sequenced Inventory of Communicative Development–Revised (Hedrick et al., 1984), a scale that contains only three questions related directly to expressive vocabulary. Second, approximately 25% of the total questions on the SICD-R (depending on a child's base or ceiling on the test) are obtained by parent report rather than by direct behavioral measures. Third, no middle-class control group was included, making it impossible to determine whether this degree of "underreporting" is unique to parents with low SES or whether the same standards of comparison would result in similar underreport on the CDIs by middle-class parents. Finally, the CDI: Words and Sentences and SICD-R scores were not obtained at the same ages.

To examine the question of SES and reliability of parent report directly, Rodrique (2001) compared parent report on a vocabulary checklist with child performance on picture book tasks designed to measure comprehension and production of those same words in 21 low-income and 23 middle-income parent–child dyads in which the children were between 18 to 32 months of age. A language checklist containing 116 words selected from the CDI: Words and Sentences form was used to examine parent report. Vocabulary comprehension was measured with a two-way forced-choice task using a book that contained 82 lifelike 8.5-inch by 11-inch photographs that represented objects, actions, and attributes. Vocabulary production was measured using a book containing 34 different 8.5-inch by 11-inch color photographs of objects or actions, and the children were asked to identify the picture. The results from this study showed no significant differences between low- and middle-income groups on either the parent report or behavioral measures of the children's language. Although these results are strikingly different from the majority of studies as of 2006, they are the first in which direct comparisons of the CDIs and behavioral measures were made. The author suggested a number of reasons that these results could have differed from earlier studies (including the fact that a majority of the families participated in Early Head Start) but noted that these results highlight the complex and multifactorial nature of the relation between SES and language development.

Clearly, considerably more research on the relation between CDI scores and other measures with children from low- and middle-SES families is needed to gain a clearer picture of the validity of the CDIs with children from low-income backgrounds. In addition, whether overreporting occurs could be influenced by the explicitness of the instructions given to parents and by whether assistance is provided in completing the form. (See the guidelines and suggestions offered at the beginning of this chapter.) Evidence is needed on the extent to which assistance can reduce under- and overreporting.

In sum, although caution should be exercised in interpreting CDI scores completed by parents with low SES, evidence to date suggests that the CDI forms can provide useful information about the language skills of this sector of the population as well. Special caution should be exercised in interpreting the CDI subscales between 8 and 12 months as some parents with lower levels of education may overestimate their child's linguistic abilities. It should also be kept in mind that some parents with lower levels of education may underreport their children's language skills on the CDI: Words and Sentences form. An ideal assessment package will never be limited to parent report or any other single measurement type.

Using the Norms with Children Who Are Learning More than One Language   Special care must also be taken when using the monolingual norms with children who are learning English and another language. The language abilities of a bilingual child may be distributed differentially across each language. Moreover, procedures using monolingual norms may not be appropriate for use with bilingual children (Anderson, 1995; Gutierrez-Clellen, 1996; Gutierrez-Clellen, Restrepo, Bedore, Peña, & Anderson, 2000). Pearson and colleagues (Pearson et al., 1993, 1993/1995, 1995; Umbel et al., 1992) proposed that a composite score derived from both languages (described in detail next) can be used in place of the standard scoring procedures. We agree with this proposal, and we have devised our scoring procedures accordingly.

A study using the CDIs and Inventarios (Marchman & Martínez-Sussmann, 2002) provided an example of the composite method. Vocabulary development was assessed for children living in Texas who heard both English and Spanish at least 12 hours per week (total number [N] = 116). Using the monolingual norms for each language, results indicated that children were delayed compared with monolinguals in each language, falling significantly below the 50th percentile as a group (p < .01) in both English and Spanish. These findings are consistent with the view that children who experience multiple language input may acquire vocabulary in each language more slowly than their monolingual peers. However, following Pearson et al. (1993, 1993/1995, 1995), a "composite" score was also derived based on the number of words that a child was reported to produce on either the CDIs or the Inventarios or on both. When the composite score was used, the bilingual children demonstrated vocabulary sizes that were comparable to monolingual peers, on average. The composite English-Spanish CDI score for evaluating bilingual children can be computed by hand or by using the CDI Scoring Program. Further studies need to be carried out to confirm the usefulness of composite scores with a bilingual population. (See the Chapter 4 section called "Validity of the Inventories" for more information about the validity of the CDIs and Inventarios when used with children who are learning English and Spanish at the same time.)

Using the Norms for the Evaluation of Older Children   Many speech-language pathologists and specialists in related fields use the CDIs with children whose chronological ages exceed the upper limits of the inventories but whose language skills are within the range seen in younger typically developing children covered by the inventory norms. Recommendations for use with these populations are discussed in Chapter 3.

3

CLINICAL AND RESEARCH APPLICATIONS

CLINICAL APPLICATIONS OF THE INVENTORIES

Many speech-language pathologists and other specialists in the early intervention field use parent report to screen children for possible language delays, to help design interventions, and to track progress in language therapy. Because parent report is not uniformly accurate, and because it is limited to selected dimensions of development, clinical management decisions concerning an individual child should never rest solely on parent input. When the CDIs (or any form of parent report) are used for diagnostic purposes, it is always best to triangulate by checking parent-reported information against direct observation and other types of assessment. Likewise, parent report may be used to confirm and elaborate conclusions based on analysis of language samples obtained in clinical settings or standardized tests. Parent report often provides a more representative sample of language than is obtained in clinical settings where spontaneous speech or test results may be influenced by the child's shyness, the unfamiliarity of the setting, and the interaction style of the examiner. For example, many young children are reluctant to talk in the presence of unfamiliar adults. Furthermore, children (like adults) rarely use all of the vocabulary words that they know in any given conversational situation. Parents are likely to have observed their children across a range of communicative situations and thus are aware of a broader range of vocabulary and other communicative acts. Parent input is therefore an important, and even an essential, ingredient in developing a profile of an individual child's communicative skills. The CDIs can contribute to the evaluation process because they are well-validated instruments with normed comparison values.

There are, however, some precautions regarding the use of the CDIs for clinical purposes. These precautions are addressed in the following sections.

Screening for Language Delay

The CDIs have considerable potential as a preliminary screening tool for delayed language. The usefulness of the instruments for screening the communication skills of infants and toddlers depends in large part on the age at which the child is screened and on the manner in which the screening is conducted. Due to the enormous variability in language and communicative development in infants and toddlers, it is virtually impossible to obtain a definite diagnosis of specific language impairment during the first 3 years of life (see Leonard, 1998; Paul, 1996, 1997; & Thal & Katich, 1996, for discussions of this issue), and identification is likely to be more solid when a child is 4 years old than 3 years old (Rescorla, 2000). Since the mid-1980s, however research on early language delay has converged on several conventions that allow practitioners to determine whether a child is at risk for persistent language impairment. Most of the studies that have used the CDIs or other parent-report instruments to study early language delay have been conducted with English-speaking children.

One common convention (known as the Delay 3 criterion, originally suggested by Rescorla, 1989) is to refer a child for further assessment and possible intervention if parents report fewer than 50 words produced or no word combinations by 24 months of age. The practice is based on the finding that these children, frequently referred to as "late talkers," may be at risk for later language impairment (Fischel, Whitehurst, Caufield, & Debaryshe, 1989; Paul, 1996; Rescorla, 1989; Rescorla & Schwartz, 1990; Rescorla & Alley, 2001; Thal & Katich, 1996). Although there is evidence that not all late talkers will have persistent language problems throughout childhood, it is accepted practice among educators and physicians to refer these children to a certified speech-language pathologist for further language assessment. Both of these screening indicators are easily obtained with the CDI: Words and Sentences form and are included on the Child Report Forms (see Appendix C).

Klee et al. (1998) reported a large number of overreferrals using the Delay 3 criterion alone; that is, some children were unnecessarily recommended for further evaluation when just the criterion was applied. However, Klee et al. (2000) significantly improved the accuracy of identification of early language delay by asking parents if they were "worried" or "had some concerns" about their child's progress in language or if their child had experienced six or more ear infections during the first 2 years of life. Klee and colleagues referred to their enhanced criterion as the Delay 3+ criterion: Fewer than 50 words *or* no word combinations AND parental concern *or* six or more ear infections during the first 2 years of life. Using the Delay 3+ criterion, a child is referred for further evaluation if he or she is 24 months old and his or her parents report any of the following:

1. The child uses fewer than 50 words and the parents are concerned about the child's language development.

2. The child uses fewer than 50 words and had six or more ear infections during the first 2 years of life.

3. The child uses more than 50 words but is not yet combining words into phrases, and the parents are concerned about the child's language development.

4. The child uses more than 50 words but is not yet combining words into phrases and had six or more ear infections during the first 2 years of life.

The Basic Information Form (Appendix B) includes similar questions, as well as questions about other factors that could be relevant to the identification of language delay (e.g., exposure to a language other than English). Thus, a screening to determine the need for further assessment following the Delay 3 or the Delay 3+ criterion is easily accomplished using the CDI: Words and Sentences form and accompanying materials.

Users should note that children who have fewer than 50 words reported on the CDI: Words and Sentences at 24 months of age fall below the 10th percentile, based on the normative data (see Tables 5.19, 5.20, and 5.21). Furthermore, as shown in Table 4.24, only 14.1% of 24-month-old girls and 14.3% of 24-month-old boys are reported not to be combining words. Thus, the original Delay 3 criterion approximates the widely used 10th percentile standard for the vocabulary production and combining indices on the CDI: Words and Sentences form.

Extension of the Delay 3 or the Delay 3+ criterion to children older than 24 months of age has not been systematically addressed in the field. Because the CDI normative tables for word production (see Tables 5.19, 5.20, and 5.21) and some of the CDI grammar subscales (e.g., Tables 5.28 through 5.30 for Examples /M3L; Tables 5.31 to 5.33 for Complexity) provide percentile scores in 5-percent increments to 30 months, a practitioner has the option of setting standards at 5% or 10% or at whatever level is desired by the user or specified by the examiner's institution or state.

A second convention for identifying language delay may be employed with children younger than 2 years of age. Research indicates that delays in both production and comprehension are more predictive of risk for persistent language impairment than delays in production only (Thal et al., 1991; Thal & Katich, 1996). Thus, for children in this age range, production vocabulary alone is not a good predictor of later language ability, and production vocabulary scores should be interpreted in the context of comprehension vocabulary and the use of gestures. That is, a child who is delayed in comprehension as well as production, and who does not make active use of gestures to assist communication, is at greater risk for persistent language delay than is a child with an expressive language delay alone.

Preliminary results in a study by Thal (2000) also suggested that rates of growth in communicative behaviors during the second year of life predict later language ability better than a static assessment of these abilities at any given age. In a study of more than 1,000 children, the rate of growth in comprehension vocabulary size measured by the CDI: Words and Gestures form at three points in time from 10 to 16 months predicted children's expressive language scores at 28 months, whereas expressive or receptive vocabulary size at any one age did not. Further research that is focused on the predictive value of trajectories of development is important for validating this finding and expanding it to languages other than English.

Labeling a child as "language delayed" and enrolling him or her in traditional language therapy burdens families psychologically and financially. Paul (1996) suggested that rather than enrolling infants and toddlers who have a delay in expressive language in traditional language therapy immediately after initial identification, children with early language delay should be reevaluated a number of times on a frequent basis. If the delay continues, then intensive, traditional intervention may be warranted. This recommendation is supported by the research findings reported by Thal (2000); it could be facilitated by using parent-report instruments such as the CDIs because they can be used to track a child's development of vocabulary and gestures over the course of several months, at the same time that other preventive interventions, such as parent education, are employed.

The CDIs are also useful for documenting the language abilities of special populations and have become more widely used for that purpose since publication of the first edition of the manual. This application includes children with autism spectrum disorders (Charman, Drew, Baird, & Baird, 2003), Down syndrome (Caselli et al., 1998; Mervis & Robinson, 2000), and Williams syndrome (Mervis & Robinson, 2000), cleft palate (Snyder & Scherer, 2004) and children born preterm (Magill-Evans & Harrison, 1999; O'Connor et al., September 12, 2002, personal communication).

Evaluation of Older Children with Language Delay

Due to clinical needs, parent-report instruments such as the CDIs are being used to assess the language of children whose chronological ages exceed the upper limits of the CDIs but whose language skills are comparable to the age range covered by the CDIs. The CDIs have many applications for evaluating older children with language impairments (e.g., for identifying areas of strength and weaknesses, for customizing interventions, for assessing response to treatment). For example, Thal, O'Hanlon, Clemmons, and Frailin (1999) demonstrated strong validity of the CDIs in two samples of children with language delay. In one sample, expressive vocabulary and grammar were assessed using the CDI: Words and Sentences form in 39- to 49-month-old children whose scores fell below the median score for 30-month-old children. In the second sample, the CDI: Words and Gestures form was used for assessing vocabulary production in 24- to 32-month-old children whose scores fell below the median score for 16-month-old children. Other researchers have reported the validity of the CDIs with older children with language delays of various etiologies including Down syndrome (Miller, Sedey, & Miolo, 1995), more general developmental delays (Yoder, Warren, & Biggar, 1997), severe cognitive impairment (McGrath, Rosmus, Canfield, Campbell, & Hennigar, 1998), and Fragile X syndrome (Jackson, 1996), as well as with children with profound hearing loss who are using cochlear implants (Mayne, Yoshinaga-Itano, Sedey, & Carey, 2000a &

2000b; Stallings, Gao, & Svirsky, 2002; Thal, DesJardin, & Eisenberg, 2006– under review). See also Chapter 4 for a review of validity research on the CDIs.

The Thal et al. (1999) findings are consonant with a suggestion made in the first edition of this manual: CDI scores for older children can only be interpreted normatively—that is, relative to other children, when the scores are at or below the median for the oldest age group in the norming samples (18 months for CDI: Words and Gestures and 30 months for CDI: Words and Sentences). As an example of the limited interpretability of scores of children older than 30 months who are above the median, consider the following scenario. Suppose the CDI: Words and Sentences Words Produced score for a 42-month-old boy is 349 words. The most appropriate reference level is always the median or 50th percentile level. Referring to Table 5.21, it would be appropriate to say that the child's productive vocabulary is equivalent to that of a median boy of age 26 months. In a sense, we are justified in saying that this child has a "language age" equivalent to the 26-month level. Suppose, however, that the same 42-month-old boy is reported to produce 660 words (i.e., near the CDI: Words and Sentences ceiling). It would not be appropriate to conclude that this child's language ability is equivalent to that of a precocious 30-month-old, nor would it be appropriate to conclude that the child is doing well. Other researchers have pointed out the psychometric limitations of age-equivalence scores for comparing children to test norms (e.g., Bishop, 1997; Lahey, 1988; Lawrence, 1992). In short, use of the CDIs to classify language level in children older than 30 months who have developmental delays is recommended only when a child's scores do not exceed the median 30-month scores on the CDI: Words and Sentences form (or the median 18-month scores when the CDI: Words and Gestures form is used). For children older than 30 months of age who have scores above the 30-month median, literal interpretation of scores requires caution to avoid serious underestimation of communicative skills resulting from ceiling effects.

Formulation of Intervention Strategies

The development of individual profiles can contribute to the identification of aspects of the child's communicative skills that may be targeted for intervention. These may include broad domains such as vocabulary production or specific ones such as particular semantic or syntactic categories. One precaution should be kept in mind when using the CDIs for this purpose. In a study of English-speaking children with developmental delays, Yoder and colleagues (1997) found that the test–retest reliability of the CDIs across a 2-week interval was excellent for the total number of words understood but marginal for individual items. The degree to which mothers were inconsistent in reporting individual comprehension of vocabulary items varied as a function of the types of words they were reporting. For example, mothers' reports tended to be more stable for nouns than for descriptive words. This suggests that the CDIs are best used to identify overall vocabulary comprehension deficits but not to identify specific words that are or are not understood for remediation. However, the case may be different with respect to production of specific words, which are usually unambiguously present or absent. Clinicians may wish to use the CDIs to identify classes of words that appear to require remediation and supplement these findings with more targeted behavioral assessments of individual words.

When individual words are a focus, the Lex2005 Database may be of interest (see http://www.sci.sdsu.edu/cdi/lexical_e.htm). This program provides month-by-month norms from 8 to 18 months (comprehension and production) of each of the 396 words and 63 gestures appearing on the CDI: Words and Gestures form and from 16 to 30 months (Words Produced) for each of the 680 words appearing on the CDI: Words and Sentences form.

Evaluation of Intervention Effects

In order to demonstrate that therapy has been effective, evidence concerning performance outside of the treatment context is essential. Parents are uniquely positioned to provide this important information; because parent report is based on a variety of contexts outside the clinic or laboratory, it can be useful for monitoring changes as a result of intervention. The CDIs have been used in clinical intervention studies to track the effects of intervention with English-speaking children who have expressive language delay (Girolametto, Pearce, & Weitzman, 1996; 1997; Girolametto, Weitzman, Wiigs, & Pearce, 1999; Robertson & Weismer, 1999) and with children who have a cleft lip and/or palate (Scherer, 1999), as well as with a child who has hearing loss and cochlear implants (Willis & Edwards, 1996).

RESEARCH APPLICATIONS

The CDIs can be administered relatively easily compared with language assessment based on language samples or standardized tests. This ease of use enables language assessment in larger samples of children than has been possible previously. In this section, we describe some research applications that follow from this capability.

Screening and Preselection of Children at Different Levels of Language Development

Researchers are often interested in studying children who are at a specific point in the language acquisition process or in tracking children from the onset of a specified milestone. A researcher interested in following the passage from first words to grammar can start with a group of children defined by age and then use one of the CDIs to determine which children meet the desired "starting point" in language development (e.g., fewer than 50 words). An example of this application may be seen in the study of naming errors as they relate to vocabulary growth (Gershkoff-Stowe & Smith, 1997).

Screening and Preselection of Children with Particular Language Characteristics or Those with Unusual Profiles

Inventories filled out by parents permit identification of late talkers (e.g., Klee et al., 1998, 2000; Rescorla, 1989; Thal & Bates, 1988), early talkers (e.g., Dale, Bates, Reznick, & Morisset, 1989; Thal, Bates, Zappia, & Oroz, 1996), or children with other specific profiles. They may also be used to select children with unusual configurations of linguistic and nonlinguistic abilities (e.g., children whose comprehension far exceeds their production; c.f. Bates, Thal, Whitesell, Fenson, & Oakes, 1989; Benedict, 1979; Snyder, Bates, & Bretherton, 1981), children who are reported to gesture extensively despite language delays (Thal et al., 1991; Thal & Tobias, 1992), and children who are surprisingly slow to produce word combinations despite their vocabulary level (Thal et al., 1996).

Matching Children on Language Skills

It is often important for researchers to ensure that groups are initially equivalent in communicative skills—for example, as when investigating the effects of specific environmental factors or intervention experiences in pre- and post-test designs. The CDIs provide researchers with an efficient means for matching children on the basis of vocabulary size, utterance length, or other relevant variables.

Examination of the Influence of Other Variables on Language Development

The CDIs permit the collection of data from relatively large samples of children in studies that assess the relation between language and global variables such as family size, SES, ethnicity, birth order, child-rearing practices, parental style, child care settings, and number of languages spoken in the home. Many of these studies have been carried out using the CDIs with English-speaking children from a variety of backgrounds (e.g., Arriaga et al., 1998; Bornstein et al., 1998, 1999; Feldman et al., 2000; Huebner, 2000; Roberts et al., 1999; Saxon, 1997). Similarly, Laakso, Poikkeus, Eklund, and Lyytinen (1999) and Lyytinen, Poikkeus, Leiwo, Ahonen, and Lyytinen (1996) used a Finnish version of the CDIs to examine the effect of parenting styles on the language development of Finnish-speaking children. Other studies have used the CDIs to examine the relation between language progress and otitis media (e.g., Feldman et al., 2003), verbal and nonverbal cognition (Dale, Dionne, Eley, & Plomin, 2000; Dionne, Dale, Boivin, & Plomin, 2003; Price, Eley, Dale, Stevenson, & Plomin, 2000), behavior and social-emotional development (Horwitz et al., 2003; Irwin, Carter, & Briggs-Gowan, 2002; Plomin, Price, Eley, Dale, & Stevenson, 2002), and language learning environment (Bornstein & Cote, 2004; Marchman & Martínez-Sussmann, 2002; Pearson et al., 1993/1995, 1995).

NON-ENGLISH VERSIONS OF THE INVENTORIES

CDIs have been developed in a number of languages other than English. A list of these versions can be found on the CDI web site at (http://www.sci.sdsu.edu/cdi/adaptations.htm). The availability of CDIs in many languages has created new opportunities for cross-linguistic studies of language development and for bilingual studies. For these reasons, the CDI Advisory Board continues to encourage the development of CDIs in additional languages, but there are some important caveats. The development of CDIs in other languages requires more than a simple translation of the original CDIs. Researchers must adapt the scales to specific cultural conventions (e.g., different gestures, games, routines, and forms of "baby talk") and, above all, to specific characteristics of the target language. For example, languages with a richer system of inflectional morphology than English require a different and more extensive assessment of grammar. Some guidelines for creating adapted versions can be found in Dale et al. (1993) and on the CDI web site (http://www.sci.sdsu.edu/cdi/guidelines_adaptations.htm).

As noted on the web site, the CDIs are copyrighted, and the creation of new adaptations of these instruments in other languages requires permission of the CDI Advisory Board. Researchers interested in creating CDI adaptations in additional languages should contact the Advisory Board, stating their interest and describing their qualifications to undertake the project. Procedures for securing approval to create adaptations are described in detail on the web site (http://www.sci.sdsu.edu/cdi/guidelines_adapatations.htm). Requests are reviewed by the Advisory Board. If permission is granted, a letter from the Advisory Board will specify any limitations on use and distribution.

4

PHASES OF THE DEVELOPMENT OF THE INVENTORIES

ORIGINS OF THE INSTRUMENTS

The CDIs have been developed across a period of more than 30 years. They originated in research by Bates and her colleagues in Rome during the early 1970s (Bates et al., 1975). Over time, as confidence in the information provided by parents grew, the measures evolved from structured interviews to questionnaire form. Reznick used a short version of the CDIs in his dissertation research (Reznick, 1982). By the late 1980s, the instruments had evolved into a set of four forms, each designed to cover a relatively narrow age range. Those instruments were the Communicative Development Questionnaire (8–12 months), the Language and Gesture Inventory (12–18 months), the Early Language Inventory (18–27 months), and the Grammatical Development Questionnaire (24–36 months). As described next, these versions were reorganized as the MacArthur CDIs, a pair of instruments for English-speaking children with reliable and valid norms that are currently widely used for clinical and research purposes (Dale, 1996; Fenson et al., 1992/1993; Fenson et al., 1994). Italian versions were developed in parallel with the English ones and were formally published a short time later (Caselli & Casadio, 1995). The CDIs have also been adapted to and normed in many other languages (see http://www.sci.sdsu.edu/cdi/adaptations_ol.htm for a list of CDI adaptations and their authors).

A Preliminary Norming Study

Portions of the early instruments exhibited excellent reliability and validity in research contexts (Bates et al., 1979; Bates, Bretherton, & Snyder, 1988; Bretherton & Bates, 1984; Dale et al., 1989; Gersten, Coster, Schneider-Rosen, Carlson, & Cicchetti, 1986; Tamis-LeMonda & Bornstein, 1989), but age-based norms had not been established. An initial norming study was conducted on these four instruments in San Diego in 1987–1988 (Fenson, Thal, & Bates, 1990). A total of 745 forms were collected on children between 9 and 36 months of age. Analyses indicated excellent developmental regularity for some of the components and less than satisfactory psychometric properties for others. For example, assessment of word comprehension did not begin until 12 months, when the median score for comprehension was already at 80 words, suggesting that testing for comprehension needed to begin several months earlier. Findings such as these provided the basis for separating the CDIs into two instruments, one for infants and one for toddlers, and both with floors and ceilings dictated by the data from the preliminary norming study. As the CDI Advisory Board became aware of the usefulness of the Inventories for older children with cognitive and/or language delay, the instrument names were changed to the CDI: Words and Gestures and the CDI: Words and Sentences, reflecting the content rather than an arbitrary and limited age range.

Two additional sources of data were used in developing the CDI forms. One was a set of word frequencies for the Early Language Inventory, based on a group of 62 20-month-old children, compiled by Reznick (1982). The other was a set of frequencies for word comprehension and production and for gestures for the Language and Gesture Inventory, based on a group of 45 children between 13–15 months of age, assembled by Bates and her students (1988).

Development of the CDI: Words and Gestures Form

The data from the norming study on the precursors of the CDIs (Fenson, Thal, & Bates, 1990) indicated that a number of aspects of communicative development are already well under way long before the end of the first year of life. Therefore, the starting age for the new form (originally called the infant form) was set at 8 months to capture the beginnings of gestural production and early word comprehension.

The CDI: Words and Gestures vocabulary list was based on the Language and Gesture Inventory list, with the following modifications. A total of 33 words that were infrequent in the Bates word comprehension data (most appearing in less than 5% of the sample) were deleted. In addition, 17 words of relatively high frequency in the 20-month frequency data, which were not present on the Language and Gesture Inventory, were added. A total of 27 words that appeared side by side as equivalent forms (e.g., *horse/pony*) were listed separately on the CDI: Words and Gestures. A new category—Sound Effects and Animal Sounds, containing items like "meow" and "vroom" that had previously been listed under the categories Animal Names and Vehicles—was added. Several categories were renamed to better reflect their content. A new "comprehension only" section consisting of common phrases was also added. Many of the phrases in this section had appeared in the Language and Gesture Inventory word list, but it seemed more appropriate to form a separate section for phrases for two reasons: 1) these combinations were highly unlikely to be in infants' production and 2) we wished to limit the vocabulary word list to single words.

The Language and Gesture Inventory also provided the initial framework for constructing the Actions and Gestures section of the new form. However, although the Actions and Gestures part of the CDI: Words and Gestures contains almost the same number of items ($n = 63$) as the Gestures Checklist on the earlier form ($n = 64$), the new form contains different items and a new organization. We examined developmental trends for each item in the first norming study (Fenson et al., 1990) and deleted or reworded those items that did not show an increasing trend across age. We also examined the 13- to 15-month-old frequency data and eliminated items with very low reported frequencies. These changes resulted in the deletion of 16 items. We added 15 new items and reorganized the former six categories into five new ones. We dropped the request that the parent indicate which actions were done in a pretend mode. Finally, in a separate section, we added a question on pretend substitutions, and we requested examples of such actions. Because this item has shown little predictive or construct validity, it has been dropped from current printings of the instrument and will not be discussed further.

Development of the CDI: Words and Sentences Form

The CDI: Words and Sentences form Part I (Vocabulary Checklist) was based on the Early Language Inventory word list, with some modifications. A total of 35 words were added, and 42 low-frequency words were dropped. Five equivalent words, which appeared side by side on the Early Language Inventory (e.g., *kitty/cat*), were listed separately.

Part II (Sentences and Grammar) was designed to assess morphological and syntactic development. Although portions of Part II were adapted from both the Early Language Inventory and the Grammatical Development Questionnaire, this section contains more new elements than any other component of the two inventories. Earlier versions of the Early Language Inventory and the Grammatical Development Questionnaire requested examples of general categories, and this request was sometimes misunderstood by the parents. Earlier versions also combined the assessment of developmental level and grammatical style, and the latter proved difficult to assess. In the new toddler form, the forced-choice recognition paradigm that had proven highly effective for assessing vocabulary and aspects of morphology in earlier forms was adapted to assess the developmental level of syntactic complexity.

Changes Reflected on Both Forms

One additional change involved the Vocabulary Checklists of both of the new forms. In the earlier versions, parents were requested to add any additional words in their child's vocabulary to the list. We dropped this request for several reasons. First, we regard the vocabulary totals as an index of a given child's vocabulary knowledge rather than an exhaustive atlas. An atlas of child vocabulary would require a list of extraordinary length. Although the present index might approach the status of an atlas for the youngest children, it becomes an increasingly smaller subset of vocabulary for older children. Indeed, the instrument's strength is that it allows assessment of individual differences in vocabulary development by making comparisons among children across a specifically defined denominator of representative words. Second, asking parents to add words increases reliance on recall, rather than recognition, and introduces individual variation in parental reporting style, thereby reducing comparability over subjects. Finally, ad hoc words are difficult to score and would not be amenable to the development of accurate norms. Although some parents will spontaneously add words that their child understands or understands and says, we recommend that these words not be included in vocabulary totals in order to ensure comparability to the normative data.

THE NORMING STUDY

Sampling Procedure

Data collection procedures varied according to sample. The following sections discuss the procedures for both the original and updated samples.

Original Sample   Data were collected for the original norming study in 1988–1989 at three sites: New Haven, Connecticut; San Diego, California; and Seattle, Washington. Funding was provided by the MacArthur Foundation to the San Diego subgroup of the MacArthur Research Network on Early Childhood Transitions, which was headed by Elizabeth Bates. The procedures for contacting parents differed across the sites. In Seattle and New Haven, public records were used to contact parents shortly after the birth of their child. Approximately 15%–20% of those contacted agreed to have their names placed in infant studies subject pools at the University of Washington (Seattle) and Yale University (Connecticut). When subsequently invited to participate in the CDI norming study, approximately 75% of the parents enrolled at each of these two sites completed and returned inventories. In San Diego, two sources were used to recruit participants. One was a subject pool comprised of individuals who had previously indicated their willingness to participate in research studies. The other was a pediatrician's mailing list. Parents were not asked in advance if they were willing to complete an inventory. Rather, they were sent a copy of the inventory with a request to complete and return it. Approximately 36% of the parents contacted did so.

Parents at each site also completed and returned a Basic Information Form, which supplied data about their child's health, the parents' educational and vocational levels, and other pertinent information. (A copy of this original version of the Basic Information Form appears in Appendix A.) At each site, parents were paid $5.00 for returning a completed inventory and Basic Information Form.

To increase the number of lower-income parents and to expand ethnic diversity, additional inventories were distributed to parents at community health centers in New Haven and San Diego. An additional 51 forms were collected in this manner.

Updated Sample   Since the publication of the original version of the manual, we have expanded and updated the norming sample with the following goals. First, we sought to increase the overall sample size, moving beyond the target of 30 boys and 30 girls per age in as many cells as possible. We set our new goal at 40 boys and 40 girls per cell, a goal that was met in 77% (17 of 22) of the cells for the CDI: Words and Gestures form and 83% (25 of 30) of the cells for the CDI Words and Sentences form.

Second, we sought to add participants to expand the age range of the CDI: Words and Gestures form, which was originally normed for children who were 8–16 months of age. However, the original norms and the data from subsequent studies showed that many of the components of the form could be extended beyond 16 months before reaching maximum values. The Spanish version of the CDI: Words and Gestures (Inventario I) also provided norming information for children who are 17–18 months of age, and we wanted to have consistency across the Spanish and English CDIs. The overlapping age ranges for the CDI: Words and Gestures form and the CDI: Words and Sentences form creates some ambiguity regarding the correct instrument to use. For some guidelines about which form to administer to best address particular research and clinical questions, see the section in Chapter 1 called "Guidelines for Choosing Between the CDI: Words and Gestures and the CDI: Words and Sentences Forms in the 16- to 18-Month Age Range." The majority of CDI: Words and Gestures forms for 17- and 18-month-old children in the updated sample were collected in Seattle, although other sites provided participants in this age range when available (see next paragraph).

A third goal of the updated norming sample was to expand the diversity of the sample, including the sites of data collection and the ethnicity and educational status of the participants. The updated sample includes the participants from the original sites (New Haven, San Diego, and Seattle), as well as new participants from several follow-up norming efforts at some of the original sites. Additional data were added from ongoing projects being conducted by members of the CDI Advisory Board. Further participants were obtained through a request on the info-childes@talkback.org mailing list. This request asked members of the child language community to share their CDI data for the purposes of updating the norming sample. The data-sharing request invited researchers to provide their first-time administrations of the CDI forms, as well as information regarding 1) exposure to a language other than English, 2) birth or health complications, 3) ethnicity, 4) birth order, and 5) maternal education. Finally, additional participants were obtained through a data collection effort that specifically targeted low-income families of African American descent from rural areas of the southern United States. This project was directed by Dr. Jana Oetting at Louisiana State University, and it was funded by the CDI Advisory Board. Data from all of these sources were compiled and screened following a consistent set of guidelines. The final updated norming sample consists of participants from Dallas, Texas; Madison, Wisconsin; New Orleans, Louisiana; New Haven, Connecticut; Providence, Rhode Island; San Diego, California; Seattle, Washington; and Storrs, Connecticut.

Medical Exclusion Criteria

In the original norming effort, forms were completed for a total of 671 infants and 1,142 toddlers. Of these 1,813 forms, 24 (12 infants and 12 toddlers) were excluded from the final sample on the basis of medical information supplied on the Basic Information Form. These included 2 children with Down syndrome, 10 children who were born 6 or more weeks prematurely, 3 children with meningitis, 3 children who had undergone extended surgical procedures, and 6 children with other serious medical problems. The most commonly reported medical problem was repeated ear infections, which was listed for 4.3% of the sample. These cases were retained in the sample. No other single problem (other than prematurity and those listed previously) was reported for more than two or three children. In the updated sample, participants were screened based on these medical exclusionary criteria prior to consideration for inclusion in the dataset. Only participants who met the guidelines established in the original effort were included.

Tables 4.1 and 4.2 show the number of girls and boys (by age) included in the original and updated norming samples for the CDI: Words and Gestures and the CDI: Words and Sentences, respectively.

Demographic Distribution of the Sample

On the basis of the information reported by the participating families, participants in the updated norming samples for the CDI: Words and Gestures form and CDI: Words and Sentences form were evaluated in terms of maternal education and ethnicity, birth order, and exposure to a second language. In the following sections, we describe the composition of the updated norming sample and compare it with the U.S. population and the original dataset.

Table 4.1. Number of children by age and sex in the original and updated norming samples (CDI: Words and Gestures)

Age in months	Original sample[a]		Updated sample	
	Girls (n)	Boys (n)	Girls (n)	Boys (n)
8	32	33	32	36
9	37	32	48	41
10	35	32	64	72
11	38	46	45	50
12	45	41	79	78
13	40	36	57	59
14	42	42	58	53
15	32	33	50	44
16	33	30	41	43
17	N/A	N/A	33	40
18	N/A	N/A	37	29
Total	**334**	**325**	**544**	**545**

[a]*Source:* Fenson, Dale, Reznick, Thal, Bates, Hartung, et al. (1992/1993) (p. 41).
Key: n = number.

Table 4.2. Number of children by age and sex in the original and updated norming samples (CDI: Words and Sentences)

Age in months	Original sample[a]		Updated sample	
	Girls (*n*)	Boys (*n*)	Girls (*n*)	Boys (*n*)
16	32	32	37	37
17	33	32	38	43
18	34	46	44	59
19	37	35	55	43
20	45	48	60	57
21	31	40	40	55
22	40	32	50	40
23	41	41	52	52
24	59	48	72	63
25	45	31	59	48
26	39	39	47	53
27	38	42	54	59
28	31	30	41	43
29	28	33	38	42
30	36	32	41	39
Total	**569**	**561**	**728**	**733**

[a]*Source:* Fenson, Dale, Reznick, Thal, Bates, Hartung, et al. (1992/1993) (p. 42).
Key: n = number.

Ethnicity and Maternal Education Table 4.3 summarizes the ethnic and educational characteristics of the updated norming sample, in relation to 2000 U.S. Census Bureau figures (see http://factfinder.census.gov/home/saff/main .html). We report educational and ethnic profiles for adults between the ages of 15 and 34 years because this subsample is a more appropriate comparison group for the parents of young children comprising our normative sample than is the U.S. population as a whole. However, these comparisons are only approximations because the information provided by the participants and the categories applied are not identical to those used by the U.S. Census Bureau (see http:// factfinder.census.gov/home/saff/main.html).

Table 4.3. Demographic profile of households in the updated norming sample compared with the U.S. population (ages 15–34 years)

Demographic characteristic	United States (%)[a]	CDI: Words and Gestures (%)	CDI: Words and Sentences (%)
Ethnicity			
White	64.2	72.9	73.7
Black	13.6	11.4	9.7
Asian	4.8	4.2	2.7
Hispanic	14.3	5.7	7.1
All others/mixed	3.2	5.7	6.9
Maternal education			
Some high school or less	15.6	6.8	8.2
High school diploma	26.2	23.6	24.1
Some college education	34.9	25.1	24.5
College diploma	23.2	44.5	43.2

[a]Derived from information available from the 2000 U.S. census (http://www.census.gov).
Instances where percentage totals vary slightly from 100 are due to rounding errors.

The ethnicity breakdown of the normative samples reflects an oversampling of Caucasian (white) participants, with African American (black) participants the second most frequently represented group. Asians, Hispanics, and those in the group "All others/mixed" each represent somewhat smaller proportions of the samples. In general, this distribution is similar to that shown by the U.S. Census figures. However, the percentage of Hispanics in the normative sample is not as high as that in the U.S. population. This is most likely the result of our requirement that children in the normative sample come from homes in which English was the primary language (see the section called "Exposure to a Second Language" for more information).

The education levels of the parents who completed the inventories are clearly well above the national average, no doubt reflecting our sampling procedures. Nevertheless, the sample had a considerable range of education levels. This diversity allowed us to examine possible effects of parents' socioeconomic level on children's language development (see the Impact of Demographic Factors on Language Outcomes section later in this chapter).

Table 4.4 compares the demographic profile of the original norming sample of the CDI (from Fenson et al., 1992/1993) with the updated sample. A comparison of these two distributions confirms that the updated sample has a substantially broader representation of ethnic groups and education levels than was observed in the original norming dataset.

Birth Order Table 4.5 shows the percentage of children by reported birth order for the CDI: Words and Gestures form and the CDI: Words and Sentences form in both the original and the updated normative samples. For both forms, most children were either first or second born, with fewer than one fifth of the children in both samples being third born or later. The birth order distributions for CDI: Words and Gestures were relatively comparable in the original and updated norming samples. However, the updated sample for the CDI: Words and Sentences includes more second-born children and notably more third-born or

Table 4.4. Demographic profile comparison of the original norms of the CDI (Fenson, Dale, Reznick, Thal, Bates, Hartung, et al., 1992/1993) and the updated norms

Demographic characteristic	Original norms (%)[a]	Revised norms (%)
Ethnicity		
White	86.9	73.3
Black	4.0	10.5
Asian	2.9	3.3
Hispanic	4.6	6.5
All others	1.6	6.4
Maternal education		
Some high school or less	4.5	7.6
High school diploma	17.9	23.9
Some college	24.3	24.8
College diploma or higher	53.3	43.8

[a]*Source:* Fenson et al. (1992/1993, p. 43).

We have slightly restructured the data here from how it appeared in the original table. In Table 4.3 of Fenson et al. (1992/1993, p. 43), there is no number provided for a "Hispanic" category; instead, that number (4.6) was mixed with the "All others" category to get 6.2.

Table 4.5. Birth order of the children in the original norms of the CDI (Fenson, Dale, Reznick, Thal, Bates, Hartung, et al., 1992/1993) and the updated norms

Birth order	CDI: Words and Gestures		CDI: Words and Sentences	
	Original (%)	Updated (%)	Original (%)	Updated (%)
First born	50.5	50.2	56.4	47.9
Second born	34.2	32.1	31.7	33.7
Third born or later	15.3	17.7	11.9	18.4

later children than in the original sample. The impact of birth order on the major language skills assessed by both CDI forms is explored later in this chapter.

Exposure to a Second Language The original normative sample was limited to children for whom English is the primary language, and that is true for the updated sample as well. However, forms were accepted for children exposed to more than one language because bilingual language environments are common for a considerable proportion of U.S. children. In the original sample, 12.2% of the parents reported that their child was exposed to a second language, although with less frequency than English. The most frequently reported second language was Spanish, which accounted for 45.6% of the total for all other languages in the bilingual sample. The other 54.4% of the bilingual sample was divided among 29 other languages. Children were not added to the updated sample if they were reported to be exposed to a substantial portion (i.e., more than 12 hours per week) of a language other than English.

DEVELOPMENTAL TRENDS IN COMMUNICATIVE SKILLS

This section provides an overview of the growth of major features of communicative development across the 8- to 30-month age span represented by the two inventories. On the basis of the updated norming data, developmental trends are presented, including the growth of vocabulary, use of gestures, and the emergence and expansion of grammar. Data are first presented for the whole sample, and then sex differences are analyzed within the sample. In the percentile tables, data are presented for both genders combined as well as for boys and girls separately.

Statistical Methods

The developmental trends were examined using the following statistical methods.

Descriptive Statistics Descriptive statistics for each section of the inventories at each month of age are displayed in this chapter. The descriptive statistics include the number of children (*n*), mean (*M*), median (*Mdn*), standard deviation (*SD*), standard error of the mean, and minimum and maximum score observed at each month. The means and standard deviations are useful for researchers or clinicians who want to know the nature of the distribution of individual scores within the normative sample. Note that in most cases the distributions of these raw scores are skewed and thus not fully described by the normal distribution and the parameters of mean and standard deviation. For this reason, additional tables are furnished that show the percentage of children who obtained scores within successive ranges (e.g., 0–100, 101–200), providing further information on the variability in these measures. A graphic representation (i.e., a figure) of the mean scores of each variable by month is also provided for many components from each CDI form. In these figures, the bars above and below each mean score represent the 95% confidence intervals, based on the standard error of the mean. The standard error of the mean, calculated as the standard deviation divided by the square root of the sample size, is an estimate of the standard deviation of the sampling distribution of means that would be expected from samples drawn from the same population. Thus, the standard error of the mean can be used as the basis for establishing confidence limits for the population at each age and comparing a new sample mean to the established norms. For example, in Figure 4.4, the mean score for vocabulary comprehension at 15 months on the CDI: Words and Gestures form is approximately 175 words. The bars above and below the mean represent the 95% confidence interval. That is, there is a 95% chance that another sample drawn from this same population would have a mean between 150 and 190 words. (These are approximations, as precise values cannot be determined from visual inspection of the graphic presentations of the actual data.) A sample with a mean outside of this range would be atypical.

Inferential Statistics   Analyses of variance (ANOVAs) were calculated to determine the effects of age and sex and their possible interaction for several key variables. On the CDI: Words and Gestures form, the measures analyzed were Phrases Understood, Words Understood, Words Produced, and Total Gestures. On the CDI: Words and Sentences, analyses were carried out for Words Produced, Examples/mean length of the three longest sentences (M3L), and Complexity. Partial eta squared (η_p^2), a measure reflecting the percent of variance accounted for, was used to determine the magnitude of each effect expressed as the percentage of variance accounted for by each significant factor. In the case of a significant interaction between age and sex, planned comparisons between males and females were conducted at each age level. Graphs depicting mean scores by age and sex also present the standard deviation for both sexes combined. Again, the mean and standard deviation are useful for examining the distribution of individual scores within the normative sample and, hence, for evaluating an individual child's score relative to this range.

Curve Fitting   Because these norms are based on cross-sectional samples, there is month-to-month sampling variability. Growth-curve modeling was used to capture the underlying pattern of increase in language skills over age. This technique, often used for models of growth (Fenson et al., 1994), uses all of the data simultaneously to show overall patterns of development and to predict scores (Burchinal & Appelbaum, 1991). Growth-curve fitting is similar to linear regression but without the restriction that the pattern over time must be a straight line. Instead, growth-curve modeling encompasses a wider range of mathematical functions. The logistic function was used for most of the present data because it is characterized by an early gradual increment, leading to a more rapid surge, and followed by a leveling off. This pattern is typically observed in the acquisition of language and in other developmental domains (Burchinal & Appelbaum, 1991).

Percentile Scores   Raw percentile scores in increments of 5, starting with the 5th percentile and ending at the 95th percentile, were calculated for both sexes combined and for boys and girls separately. In addition, the 99th percentile values are also provided to demarcate the top of the distribution. Using these percentile scores, fitted scores were then calculated using the previously described growth-curve techniques. Fitted percentile scores were calculated for Phrases Understood, Words Understood, Words Produced, Total Gestures, Early Gestures, and Later Gestures on the CDI: Words and Gestures form and for Words Produced, Complexity, Examples/M3L, Word Forms and Word Endings/Part 2 on the CDI: Words and Sentences form. The growth curves for the 90th, 75th, 50th, 25th, and 10th percentiles for these variables are also depicted graphically in Chapter 5. Standard scores are not provided because of the skew of the distributions. We believe that percentile scores best capture the language abilities of children relative to other children of the same age.

Developmental Trends in Communicative Development Specific to the CDI: Words and Gestures Form

Developmental trends in communicative development were calculated for each of the components of the CDI: Words and Gestures. These trends are detailed next.

First Signs of Understanding   The First Signs of Understanding section was included in the CDI: Words and Gestures form to tap rudimentary signs of understanding in very young infants who do not yet show evidence of specific word comprehension. Table 4.6 presents the percentage of children at each age for whom their parents reported 0–1, 2, or 3 *yes* responses. The results indicated that approximately 75% of the children were reported to exhibit all three of these behaviors at 8 months of age. This value increased to more than 80% at 10 months and more than 95% by 11 months. Virtually all of the 12-month-olds were reported to exhibit each of these behaviors.

These early signs of language comprehension were clearly typical of the vast majority of the children across the age range sampled. Similarly high levels were observed in the original norming sample and the data for the Spanish Inventario I. One might question the diagnostic value of these questions because so many children are at the ceiling from an early age. In our experience, this section is useful for parents whose children are very young or are developing quite slowly for their age. The beginning of the scale gives these parents confidence that their children are "in the ballpark" before they proceed to the more demanding items contained in the subsequent sections. Moreover, chil-

Table 4.6. Percent of children with 0–1, 2, or 3 *yes* responses in First Signs of Understanding (CDI: Words and Gestures)

Age in months	Girls Number of *yes* responses			Boys Number of *yes* responses		
	0–1	2	3	0–1	2	3
8	3.1	18.8	78.1	8.4	16.7	75.0
9	0	10.4	89.6	2.4	12.2	85.4
10	6.2	7.8	85.9	1.4	15.3	83.3
11	0	2.2	97.8	0	2.0	98.0
12	0	0	100.0	0	1.3	98.7
13	1.8	0	98.2	0	3.3	96.6
14	0	5.2	94.8	3.8	1.9	94.3
15	0	6.0	94.0	0	0	100.0
16	4.9	0	95.1	0	2.3	97.7
17	3.0	0	97.0	2.5	2.5	95.0
18	0	0	100.0	0	0	100.0

dren who show none of these early signs of understanding are likely to be at risk for some form of developmental delay.

Phrases Understood Figure 4.1 shows the mean number of common phrases reported as understood by month. The developmental trend is monotonic (i.e., the number of phrases reported as understood increases regularly across the age range). The confidence intervals indicate relatively constant variance throughout the age period.

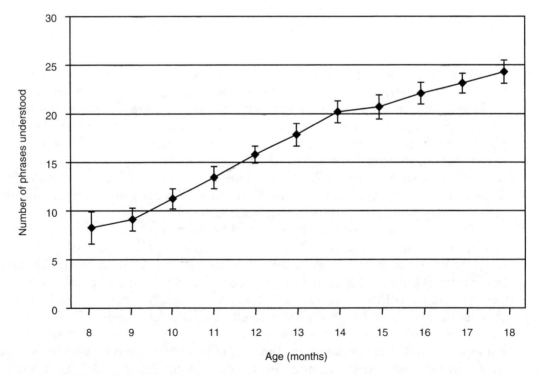

Figure 4.1. Mean Phrases Understood (CDI: Words and Gestures) scores by age in months. (*Note:* Bars above and below each mean score represent the 95% confidence intervals.)

Table 4.7. Descriptive statistics for Phrases Understood (CDI: Words and Gestures)

Age in months	n	M	Mdn	SD	Standard error of the mean	Minimum	Maximum[a]
8	68	8.3	6.0	6.8	0.8	0	26
9	89	9.1	9.0	5.6	0.6	0	27
10	136	11.2	11.0	6.2	0.5	0	27
11	95	13.4	13.0	5.6	0.6	0	28
12	157	15.8	15.0	5.5	0.4	4	28
13	116	17.8	18.0	6.4	0.6	0	28
14	111	20.2	21.0	6.0	0.6	5	28
15	94	20.7	22.0	6.1	0.6	5	28
16	84	22.1	24.0	5.1	0.6	7	28
17	73	23.1	24.0	4.3	0.5	8	28
18	66	24.3	26.0	4.9	0.6	8	28

[a]Maximum score possible = 28.

Key: n = number; *M* = mean; *Mdn* = median; *SD* = standard deviation.

More complete descriptive statistics for the number of phrases understood are presented in Table 4.7. As in the original normative sample (see Figure 4.1 on p. 47 of Fenson et al., 1992/1993), understanding of phrases was reported as early as 8 or 9 months of age, with a steady increase in the number of items reported across the CDI: Words and Gestures age range. As would be expected, the standard deviations are quite substantial at each monthly interval, especially in the younger age ranges, indicating that there is considerable variation in comprehension, particularly among younger children.

Table 4.8 further highlights the variation in the number of phrases that were reported to be understood by 8- to 18-month-old English-speaking children. This table presents the percentage of children with 0, 1–10, 11–20, and 21–28 phrases understood at each monthly interval. At virtually all ages, some children were reported to understand very few phrases, whereas other children approached or reached the ceiling level of 28 phrases. By 10 months, however, almost half of the children were reported to understand 11–20 of the phrases listed. By 14 months, approximately half (51.4%) of the children understood

Table 4.8. Percentage of children with Phrases Understood (CDI: Words and Gestures) scores falling in four successive ranges

	Phrases Understood scores[a]			
Age in months	0	1–10	11–20	21–28
8	5.9	63.2	25.0	5.9
9	2.2	65.2	29.2	3.4
10	2.2	44.1	44.9	8.8
11	1.1	28.4	60.0	10.5
12	0	18.5	58.0	23.6
13	0.9	13.8	50.0	35.3
14	0	7.2	41.4	51.4
15	0	10.6	33.0	56.4
16	0	1.2	35.7	63.1
17	0	1.4	15.1	83.6
18	0	4.5	10.6	84.8

[a]Maximum score possible = 28.

21–28 of the phrases. By 18 months, almost all of the children in the sample (84.8%) understood the majority of the phrases (i.e., 21–28 phrases).

Figure 4.2 depicts the mean number of phrases understood for boys and girls separately at each month. A 2 (sex) × 11 (age) between-subjects ANOVA on number of phrases understood yielded significant main effects for age $F(10, 1067) = 82.8$, $p < .001$, and sex, $F(1, 1067) = 11.9$, $p < .001$, but no significant age by sex interaction, $F(10, 1067) = 0.5$, ns (F stands for "Fisher's F ratio"; p stands for "probability"; ns stands for "nonsignificant"). Estimates of the variance accounted for (η_p^2) indicated that age accounted for 43% of the variance and sex accounted for approximately 1% of the variance. These findings make it clear that many young infants understand a considerable number of phrases and demonstrate consistent growth in this skill through 18 months of age. Girls display a significant, but slight, advantage in the comprehension of phrases throughout the age range. It should be noted that appropriate responses to these familiar phrases occur in context, often accompanied by familiar gestures. Thus, understanding of the phrases listed on the CDI: Words and Gestures should not be equated with genuine comprehension of multiword combinations, which would be expected to emerge later. The percentiles by age and sex for this measure are presented in Tables 5.1, 5.2, and 5.3 in Chapter 5.

Starting to Talk   The Starting to Talk section contains two questions: One asks how often the child imitates words or parts of sentences, and the other asks how often the child names or labels things. For purposes of analy-

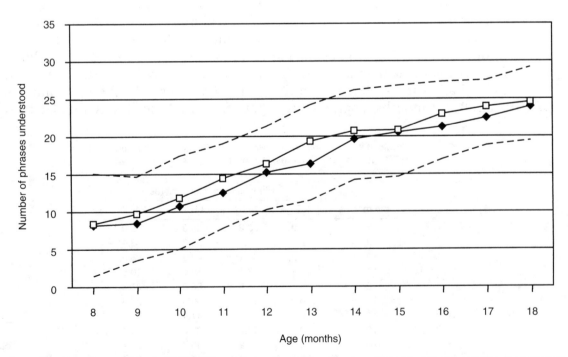

Figure 4.2.   Mean Phrases Understood (CDI: Words and Gestures) scores by age and sex. (*Note:* The dashed lines represent ±1 standard deviation for the sexes combined.) (*Key:* ◆ = boys; □ = girls.)

sis, *often* and *sometimes* were combined to form a "behavior present" category, to be contrasted with a "behavior-not-present" category (based on the frequency of *never* responses). Figure 4.3 shows the percentage of children at each month with *yes* (behavior present) responses for Imitation and Labeling, and Table 4.9 presents the percentage of boys and girls with affirmative responses. Although both of these behaviors showed an increasing developmental trend, Imitation was reported to be more common at each month than Labeling. Growth in the number of children reported to label objects did not begin until 10–11 months of age. Differences between boys and girls for Imitation were evaluated with a 2 (sex) × 11 (age) between-subjects ANOVA. As expected, there was a significant main effect of age, $F(10, 1067) = 23.8$, $p < .0001$. However, there was neither a significant main effect of sex, $F(1, 1067) = 2.6$, *ns*, nor a significant sex by age interaction, $F(10, 1067) = .73$, *ns*. Thus, age accounted for the vast majority of the developmental change ($\eta_p^2 = 18.2\%$), with this aspect of early communication showing a similar upward trend throughout this period for both boys and girls. For Labeling, analyses revealed significant main effects of age, $F(10, 1067) = 42.1$, $p < .0001$, and sex, $F(1, 1067) = 10.2$, $p < .001$, but no significant age by sex interaction, $F(10, 1067) = 1.6$, *ns*. Age accounted for approximately 28% of the variance, sex for approximately 0.9%. Thus, the tendency to label objects increases across this developmental range, and girls demonstrated a very slight advantage across the age period.

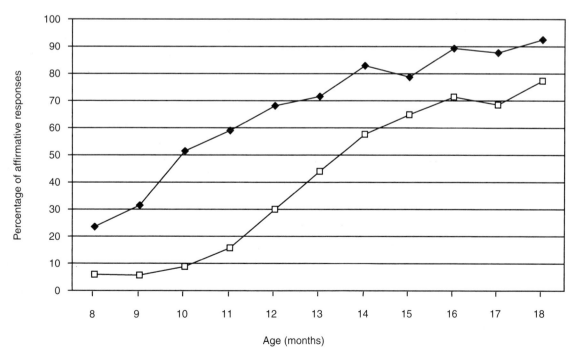

Figure 4.3. Percentage of children with affirmative (*sometimes* or *often*) responses for Imitation and Labeling in Starting to Talk (CDI: Words and Gestures) by age in months. (*Key:* ◆ = imitation; □ = labeling.)

Table 4.9. Percentage of children with affirmative (*sometimes* or *often*) responses for Imitation and Labeling in Starting to Talk (CDI: Words and Gestures)

| | Starting to Talk | | | |
| | Imitation | | Labeling | |
Age in months	Girls	Boys	Girls	Boys
8	25.0	22.2	6.3	5.6
9	35.4	26.8	8.3	2.4
10	50.0	52.8	15.6	2.8
11	64.4	54.0	17.8	14.0
12	74.7	61.5	39.2	20.5
13	78.9	64.4	52.6	35.6
14	81.0	84.9	58.6	56.6
15	78.0	79.5	60.0	70.5
16	92.7	86.0	75.6	67.4
17	84.8	90.0	84.8	55.0
18	94.6	89.7	78.4	75.9

Vocabulary Checklist (Words Understood) Based on the responses on the Vocabulary Checklist, Figure 4.4 presents the mean number of words understood by age in months. This figure shows a gradual, monotonically increasing trend in the number of words that informants reported children understood from 9 through 18 months of age. The level of vocabulary comprehension observed in the present sample of children is generally comparable to the original

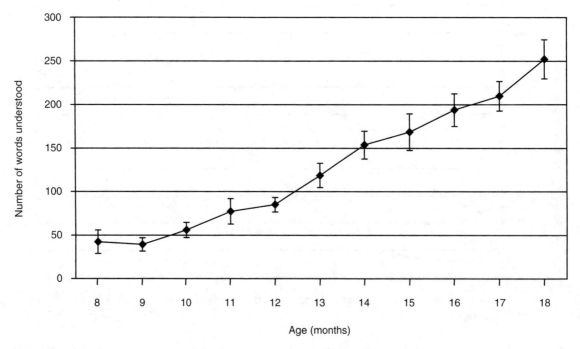

Figure 4.4. Mean Words Understood (CDI: Words and Gestures) scores by age in months. (*Note:* Bars above and below each mean score represent the 95% confidence intervals.)

Table 4.10. Descriptive statistics for Words Understood (CDI: Words and Gestures)

Age in months	n	M	Mdn	SD	Standard error of the mean	Minimum	Maximum[a]
8	68	42.3	21.0	55.4	6.7	0	261
9	89	39.3	25.0	35.7	3.8	0	177
10	136	55.8	39.5	51.3	4.4	0	280
11	95	77.1	55.0	71.7	7.4	6	396
12	157	84.9	74.0	52.5	4.2	7	263
13	116	118.7	112.0	76.6	7.1	0	395
14	111	153.6	150.0	84.8	8.0	3	393
15	94	168.4	151.5	102.2	10.5	12	396
16	84	193.6	177.0	86.7	9.5	40	396
17	73	209.7	210.0	73.1	8.6	9	340
18	66	252.0	268.0	90.7	11.2	31	395

[a]Maximum score possible = 396.

Key: n = number; *M* = mean; *Mdn* = median; *SD* = standard deviation.

sample (see Figure 4.3 on p. 48 of Fenson et al., 1992/1993), with the average number of words understood continuing to increase between 16 and 18 months of age.

Table 4.10 presents more complete descriptive statistics for the number of words understood by age in months. Mean scores were below 50 words at the 2 earliest months and increased steadily thereafter to a mean of more than 200 words at 17 and 18 months. At 8, 9, 10, and 13 months, reports indicated that at least one child did not understand any words. No child reached the ceiling of 396 words until 15 months, although at least one child approached that level at both 13 and 14 months. There is considerable variation in vocabulary comprehension levels across the age range, especially in the later months. The fitted percentile scores for this measure can be found in Tables 5.4, 5.5., and 5.6 in Chapter 5.

Variability in the number of words understood can be further seen in Table 4.11. This table presents the percentage of children at each age with reported

Table 4.11. Percentage of children with Words Understood (CDI: Words and Gestures) scores falling in four successive ranges

	Words Understood[a]			
Age in months	0–100	101–200	201–300	301–396
8	88.2	7.4	4.4	0
9	89.9	10.1	0	0
10	85.3	12.5	2.2	0
11	77.9	17.9	1.1	3.2
12	70.7	26.1	3.2	0
13	43.1	45.7	7.8	3.4
14	30.6	40.5	21.6	7.2
15	30.9	35.1	18.1	16.0
16	13.1	45.2	29.8	11.9
17	8.2	32.9	49.3	9.6
18	7.6	21.2	36.4	34.8

[a] Maximum score possible = 396.

comprehension scores falling in four successive vocabulary ranges: 0–100, 101–200, 201–300, and 301–396 words. Most children in the sample fell in the lowest range between 8 and 12 months, whereas more than one third of the children reached the highest levels at 18 months. There was a substantive increase in the proportion of children falling in the upper levels for number of words understood between 16 and 18 months of age, highlighting the significant developmental growth in vocabulary comprehension that is observed in the age range.

The number of words understood by boys and girls at each age is shown in Figure 4.5. These scores were evaluated with a 2 (sex) × 11 (age) between-subjects ANOVA. There was a significant main effect of age, $F(10, 1067) = 86.9$, $p < .0001$ and sex, $F(1, 1067) = 19.0$, $p < .0001$, however, the interaction between sex and age was not significant, $F(10, 1067) = .84$, ns. Age accounted for the vast majority ($\eta_p^2 = 44.9\%$) of the variance, with sex accounting for only 1.7%. Thus, for both boys and girls vocabulary comprehension showed an upward trend throughout this period, with girls showing a consistent, albeit slight, advantage at all months.

Vocabulary Checklist (Words Produced)   Figure 4.6 presents the mean number of reported words produced (for both sexes combined) by age in months. This figure shows a gradual, monotonically increasing trend from 8 to 18 months. The mean score for vocabulary production did not exceed 20 words until 14

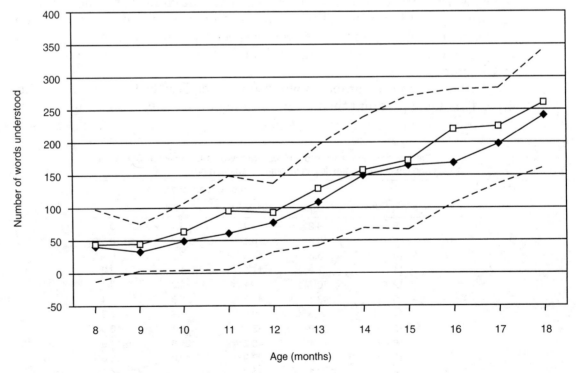

Figure 4.5.   Mean Words Understood (CDI: Words and Gestures) scores by age and sex. (*Note:* The dashed lines represent ±1 standard deviation for the sexes combined.) (*Key:* ◆ = boys; □ = girls.)

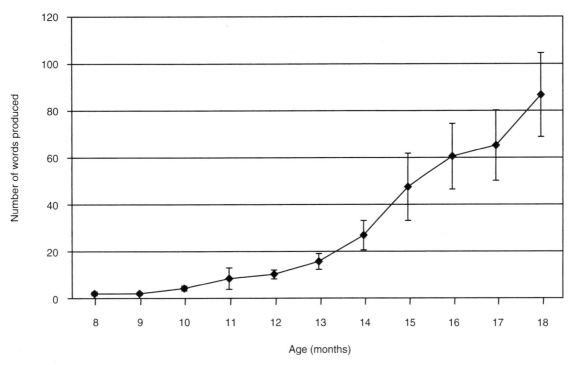

Figure 4.6. Mean Words Produced (CDI: Words and Gestures) scores by age in months. (*Note:* Bars above and below each mean score represent the 95% confidence intervals.)

months, yet by 18 months, the average child was reported to produce approximately 85 words. The confidence intervals suggest relatively narrow ranges of scores for young infants but quite substantial variation in the later months. The growth trend is slightly lower, although generally comparable to that reported by Fenson et al. (1992/1993) based on the original norming sample (see Figure 4.4 on p. 49 in Fenson et al., 1992/1993). As with the number of words understood, there is considerable growth in reported word production in the 16- to 18-month period.

Complete descriptive statistics for the number of words produced are presented in Table 4.12. At all months, the standard deviations are comparable to or larger than their respective means, highlighting the wide variability in the distribution of scores for vocabulary production across the age range. This phenomenon is also seen in the original English CDI sample (see Figure 4.4 on p. 49 of Fenson et al., 1992/1993). Percentile tables are presented in Tables 5.7, 5.8, and 5.9 of Chapter 5.

Table 4.13 further illustrates the variability within the population in the number of words produced. As would be expected, at the younger months, a large majority of the children were reported to produce very few words. For instance, at 8 months of age, informants reported that 51.5% of the sample did not yet produce any words, and 42.6% of the sample was reported to produce between 1 and 10 words. With development, however, reports indicated that fewer children produced no words at all, and several of the 12-month-olds used more than 50 words. By 18 months of age, all of the children were reported to

Table 4.12. Descriptive statistics for Words Produced (CDI: Words and Gestures)

Age in months	n	M	Mdn	SD	Standard error of the mean	Minimum	Maximum[a]
8	68	2.0	.0	3.1	0.4	0	13
9	89	2.0	1.0	2.6	0.3	0	13
10	136	4.2	3.0	6.0	0.5	0	53
11	95	8.4	3.0	22.7	2.3	0	213
12	157	10.0	5.0	12.0	1.0	0	66
13	116	15.7	11.0	18.6	1.7	0	107
14	111	26.8	17.0	33.0	3.1	0	193
15	94	47.4	18.0	70.1	7.2	0	376
16	84	60.5	40.0	64.6	7.0	0	347
17	73	65.2	39.0	64.4	7.5	0	293
18	66	86.7	59.0	72.7	9.0	4	327

[a]Maximum score possible = 396.

Key: n = number; M = mean; Mdn = median; SD = standard deviation.

produce at least one word, and 34.8% were producing more than 100 words. No child in the sample approached the ceiling value of 396 words.

Figure 4.7 presents the mean number of words produced by age and sex. Results of a 2 (sex) × 11 (age) between-subjects ANOVA for vocabulary production revealed a significant main effect of age, $F(10, 1067) = 48.1$, $p < .0001$, a significant main effect of sex, $F(1, 1067) = 29.0$, $p < .0001$ and a significant age by sex interaction, $F(10, 1067) = 4.5$, $p < .0001$. Estimates of the practical significance of these effects indicated that age accounted for 31% of the variance, sex accounted for 2.6% of the variance, and age by sex interaction accounted for approximately 4% of the variance. Because of the significant interaction term, planned comparisons were conducted contrasting boys and girls at each age level. These comparisons indicated that girls were reported to produce significantly more words than boys only at 16 and 18 months of age ($p < .05$). Thus, reported word production is characterized by an upward trend through 18 months of age, with girls producing significantly more words than boys in the later age

Table 4.13. Percentage of children with Words Produced (CDI: Words and Gestures) scores falling in six successive ranges

Age in months	Words Produced[a]					
	0	1–10	11–20	21–50	51–100	>100
8	51.5	42.6	5.9	0	0	0
9	43.8	55.1	1.1	0	0	0
10	29.4	59.6	10.3	0	0.7	0
11	16.8	63.2	12.6	6.3	0	1.1
12	13.4	52.2	18.5	14.6	1.3	0
13	7.8	40.5	28.4	18.1	3.4	1.7
14	6.3	29.7	21.6	29.7	9.0	3.6
15	6.4	23.4	25.5	19.1	12.8	12.8
16	2.4	11.9	16.7	26.2	25.0	17.9
17	1.4	11.0	13.7	31.5	16.4	26.0
18	0	6.1	10.6	25.8	22.7	34.8

[a]Maximum score possible = 396.

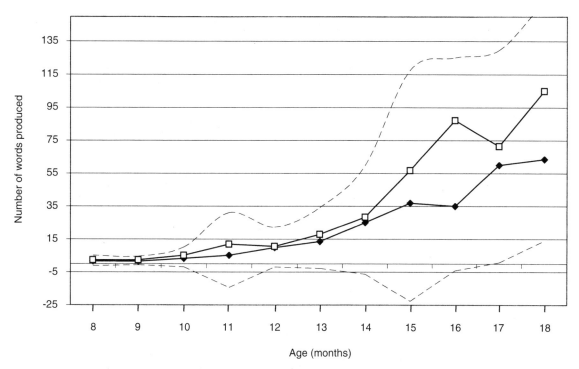

Figure 4.7.   Mean Words Produced (CDI: Words and Gestures) scores by age and sex. (*Note:* The dashed lines represent ±1 standard deviation for the sexes combined.) (*Key:* ◆ = boys; □ = girls.)

period. The relatively small amount of variance accounted for by sex suggests that the effect of sex is small compared to the general developmental growth that occurs during this period.

In general, these developmental functions are concordant with reports in the literature concerning time of onset and subsequent developmental course of language comprehension and production from 8 to 18 months of age (Bates et al., 1988; Benedict, 1979; Nelson, 1973; Rescorla, 1989, 1991). One exception may be the relatively high levels of word comprehension reported for children in the top 10% of the distribution at 8 to 10 months (see Table 5.4). These estimates (106 words at 9 months and 134 words at 10 months) exceed all prior estimates reported in the child language literature. We suspect that some parents may have adopted a different, more liberal definition of *understands* than we intended. By contrast, the range of variation observed for early word production falls within the range suggested by observational studies of first words in this same age period.

Actions and Gestures (Total Gestures)   Figure 4.8 shows the mean of the total number of gestures used (maximum = 64) reported for both sexes combined at each month. Mean gesture usage increased monotonically across the 8- to 18-month age span. The variation remained relatively constant throughout the age period.

Table 4.14 provides further descriptive statistics for the total number of gestures used as a function of age. Total scores averaged 10.7 gestures at 8 months and increased to 47.8 gestures by 18 months. These means are very

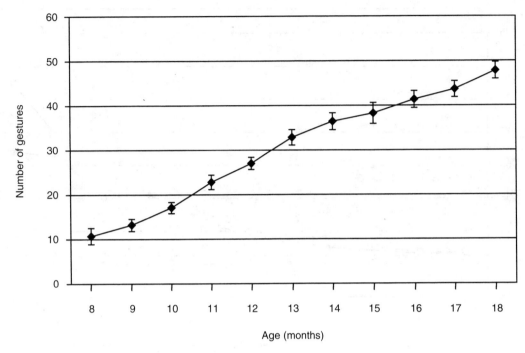

Figure 4.8. Mean Total Gestures (CDI: Words and Gestures) scores by age in months. (*Note:* Bars above and below each mean score represent the 95% confidence intervals.)

similar to those reported in the original English-speaking sample (see Figure 4.5 on p. 51 of Fenson et al., 1992/1993). As with the other measures, the range of scores was considerable throughout the age range. The percentile tables for this measure are Tables 5.10, 5.11, and 5.12 in Chapter 5.

The variability in the total number of gestures produced can be further examined in Table 4.15. At the youngest ages (8–10 months), reports showed that at least one child at each age level did not produce any gestures, whereas a few children had scores representing half of the possible items. From 16 to 18

Table 4.14. Descriptive statistics for Total Gestures (CDI: Words and Gestures)

Age in months	n	M	Mdn	SD	Standard error of the mean	Minimum	Maximum[a]
8	68	10.7	8.5	7.6	0.9	0	34
9	89	13.2	13.0	6.6	0.7	0	38
10	136	17.1	17.0	7.4	0.6	0	49
11	95	22.8	22.0	8.0	0.8	10	42
12	156	27.0	27.0	8.7	0.7	0	58
13	113	32.8	33.0	9.3	0.9	9	61
14	110	36.4	36.0	10.0	1.0	14	59
15	93	38.3	40.0	11.5	1.2	3	63
16	83	41.3	42.0	8.7	1.0	21	58
17	73	43.7	45.0	7.9	0.9	24	61
18	66	47.8	48.5	7.6	0.9	32	62

[a]Maximum score possible = 63.

Key: n = number; M = mean; Mdn = median; SD = standard deviation.

Table 4.15. Percentage of children with Total Gestures (CDI: Words and Gestures) scores falling in seven successive ranges

Age in months	Total Gestures[a]						
	0	1–10	11–20	21–30	31–40	41–50	51–63
8	2.9	57.4	29.4	8.8	1.5	0	0
9	3.4	36.0	51.7	7.9	1.1	0	0
10	0.7	15.4	57.4	22.1	3.7	0.7	0
11	0	1.1	44.2	36.8	15.8	2.1	0
12	1.9	1.3	16.0	49.4	25.0	5.8	0.6
13	0	.9	8.8	30.1	38.9	18.6	2.7
14	0	0	4.5	23.6	37.3	25.5	9.1
15	0	1.1	7.5	15.1	30.1	33.3	12.9
16	0	0	0	14.5	27.7	43.4	14.5
17	0	0	0	6.8	26.0	43.8	23.3
18	0	0	0	0	18.2	45.5	36.4

[a]Maximum score possible = 63.

months, several children approached the ceiling score of 63 gestures, yet a few children remained in the range of fewer than 20 gestures.

The mean of the total number of gestures produced by boys and girls at each age is plotted in Figure 4.9. These scores were evaluated using a 2 (sex) × 11 (age) between-subjects ANOVA. There was a significant main effect of age, $F(10, 1060) = 186.5$, $p < .0001$, and a significant main effect of sex, $F(1, 1060) = 30.4$, $p < .001$. The age by sex interaction was not significant, $F(10, 1060) = 1.6$, ns.

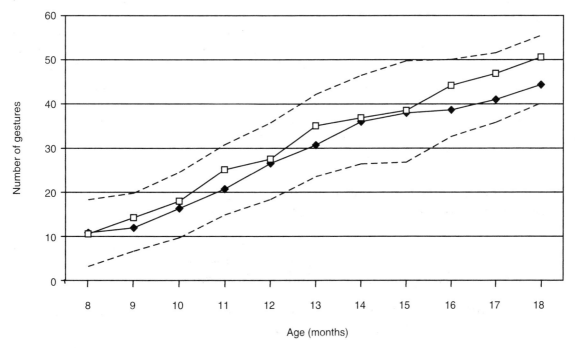

Figure 4.9. Mean Total Gestures (CDI: Words and Gestures) scores by age and sex. (*Note:* The dashed lines represent ±1 standard deviation for the sexes combined.) (*Key:* ◆ = boys; □ = girls.)

Table 4.16. Descriptive statistics for Early Gestures and Later Gestures (CDI: Words and Gestures)

Age in months	n	Early Gestures[a]			Later Gestures[b]		
		M	Mdn	SD[c]	M	Mdn	SD
8	68	28.4	28.6	16.9	11.0	7.0	10.6
9	89	36.6	38.1	16.0	12.7	11.6	10.0
10	136	43.8	42.9	13.9	18.3	16.3	12.2
11	95	48.8	47.6	12.9	29.1	25.6	15.0
12	156	54.8	57.1	13.3	36.0	34.9	15.9
13	113	60.9	61.9	11.1	46.7	46.5	18.2
14	110	63.5	66.7	13.6	53.7	51.2	19.0
15	93	64.4	66.7	13.1	57.6	58.1	21.7
16	83	65.9	66.7	11.1	63.9	65.1	16.9
17	73	69.7	71.4	11.5	67.5	69.8	14.5
18	66	72.6	76.2	10.1	75.6	75.6	14.4

[a] For Early Gestures, mean and median scores are reported as a percentage of 21 opportunities.
[b] For Later Gestures, mean and median scores are reported as a percentage of 43 opportunities.
Key: n = number; *M* = mean; *Mdn* = median; *SD* = standard deviation.

Age accounted for approximately 64% of the variance, and sex accounted for 2.8% of the variance. As graphed in Figure 4.9, girls tended to maintain a statistical edge over boys, but the magnitude of the difference in the average number of gestures for the two sexes was consistently quite small relative to the variation within each sex and across the developmental period.

Table 4.16 presents descriptive statistics for two gesture subcategories, Early Gestures (the sum of Sections A and B of the Actions and Gestures section) and Later Gestures (the sum of Sections C through E of the Actions and Gestures sections). Consistent with findings from the original norming study, items comprising the Early Gestures subsection are more likely to be reported than items in the Later Gestures sections prior to 15 months of age. On average, children were reported to produce half of the Early Gestures by 12 months of age but half of the Later Gestures at 14 months of age. By 18 months, informants reported that children produced more than 70% of the gestures in both sections. As with the other measures, there is considerable variation in the number of gestures reported in each of these two subsections throughout the age range sampled.

Developmental Trends in Communicative Development Specific to the CDI: Words and Sentences Form

Developmental trends in communicative development for each component of CDI: Words and Sentences are presented in this section in the order that they appear on that form and on the Child Report Form.

Vocabulary Checklist (Words Produced) Figure 4.10 presents the mean number of words produced for both sexes combined for children 16–30 months of age. The scores reflect a gradual monotonic trend, with relatively stable variation across the age range. The average number of words produced reported by

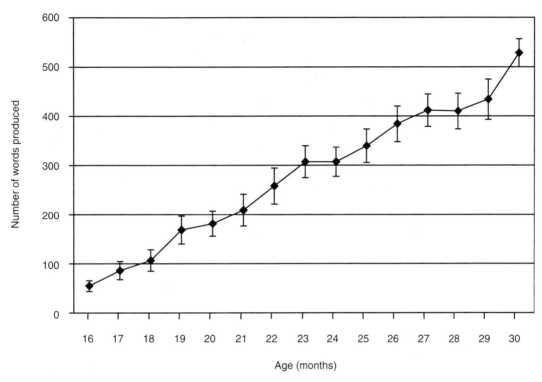

Figure 4.10. Mean Words Produced (CDI: Words and Sentences) scores by age in months. (*Note:* Bars above and below each mean score represent the 95% confidence intervals.)

parents was approximately 60 at 16 months, increasing to more than 500 words by 30 months.

Table 4.17 provides complete descriptive information about the number of words produced by children at each month. These results highlight the variability across the entire age range, with scores spanning a wide range of values at each age. Even in the upper portion of this age span, there were children reported to be using well under 40 words. At the same time, at all months excepting the two lowest, one or more children were credited with more than 500 words. The pattern of reported vocabulary production was generally comparable to the findings from the original norming study (see Figure 4.7 on p. 54 in Fenson et al., 1992/1993).

Comparing the mean number of words produced for 16-, 17-, and 18-month-olds on CDI: Words and Sentences with the means for the same index on CDI: Words and Gestures (see Tables 4.17 and 4.12, respectively), we note that the means were comparable at 16 months, but considerably higher at 17 and 18 months for the children in the CDI: Words and Sentences sample. Although this finding could be a consequence of the composition of the two different norming samples, it could also result from the fact that the CDI: Words and Sentences Vocabulary Checklist contains more words (680) than the CDI: Words and Gestures Vocabulary Checklist (396), providing more words that may be in a child's expressive vocabulary. The first possibility seems unlikely given the similarity in demographic characteristics across the two samples (see Table 4.3).

Table 4.17. Descriptive statistics for Words Produced (CDI: Words and Sentences)

Age in months	n	M	Mdn	SD	Standard error of the mean	Minimum	Maximum[a]
16	74	58.9	42.5	59.1	6.9	6	357
17	81	86.2	57.0	84.0	9.3	7	488
18	103	107.1	72.0	110.5	10.9	0	508
19	98	167.0	125.0	138.9	14.0	3	580
20	117	181.3	148.0	134.5	12.4	3	544
21	95	208.1	159.0	157.1	16.1	3	599
22	90	256.6	263.5	166.9	17.6	8	600
23	104	313.4	309.0	162.4	15.9	25	638
24	135	307.3	306.0	171.0	14.7	7	668
25	107	338.2	373.0	178.1	17.2	23	672
26	100	382.5	412.0	180.7	18.1	26	662
27	113	408.2	429.0	176.2	16.6	17	678
28	84	414.1	431.0	158.4	17.3	2	674
29	80	433.1	462.0	174.7	19.5	33	680
30	80	518.6	561.0	125.2	14.0	117	675

[a]Maximum score possible = 680.

Key: n = number; *M* = mean; *Mdn* = median; *SD* = standard deviation.

The second possibility seems more plausible, particularly because a similar result was observed in the original norming study at the single overlapping age point (i.e., 16 months). Nevertheless, the discrepancies in absolute scores across the two forms serve as reminders that the checklists provide indices of children's relative levels and thus provide a means for comparing individual differences among children only on a particular form (not across the two forms).

The variability in the number of words produced is further illustrated in Table 4.18 by the proportion of children at each age who fall within seven vocabulary ranges. At 16 months, the reports showed that more than 80% of the sample produced between 0 and 100 words, and only one child produced more than 300

Table 4.18. Percentage of children with Words Produced (CDI: Words and Sentences) scores falling in seven successive ranges

Age in months	Words Produced[a]						
	0–100	101–200	201–300	301–400	401–500	501–600	601–680
16	83.8	13.5	1.4	1.4	0	0	0
17	71.6	18.5	7.4	1.2	1.2	0	0
18	60.2	25.2	6.8	3.9	2.9	1.0	0
19	42.9	24.5	12.2	13.3	4.1	3.1	0
20	38.5	21.4	21.4	9.4	7.7	1.7	0
21	30.5	28.4	13.7	12.6	9.5	5.3	0
22	25.6	18.9	13.3	20.0	14.4	7.8	0
23	10.6	18.3	20.2	21.2	12.5	12.5	4.8
24	15.6	14.8	18.5	19.3	15.6	12.6	3.7
25	13.1	17.8	8.4	18.7	23.4	13.1	5.6
26	9.0	12.0	15.0	9.0	21.0	25.0	9.0
27	3.5	12.4	14.2	14.2	16.8	25.7	13.3
28	2.4	10.7	9.5	20.2	22.6	22.6	11.9
29	5.0	8.8	10.0	15.0	21.3	16.3	23.8
30	0	1.3	3.8	15.0	12.5	36.3	31.3

[a]Maximum score possible = 680.

words. By 19 months, a majority of the children were reported to produce more than 100 words, although production vocabularies that were larger than 400 words were still relatively rare. At 24 months, considerable variation was still evident, with an almost even distribution across all vocabulary levels. By 30 months, however, slightly more than 80% of the children were reported to produce more than 400 words. At the same time, reports for a few children indicated production vocabularies of fewer than 200 words.

The mean number of words produced for girls and boys at each age level is depicted in Figure 4.11. Vocabulary production totals were analyzed with a 2 (sex) × 15 (age) between-subjects ANOVA. This analysis yielded significant main effects for age, $F(14, 1431) = 76.4$, $p < .0001$, and sex, $F(1, 1431) = 40.5$, $p < .0001$, but a nonsignificant age by sex interaction, $F(14, 1431) = 0.8$, *ns*. Age accounted for approximately 43% of the variance, whereas sex accounted for only approximately 3% of the variance. As seen in Figure 4.11, mean differences contributing to a significant advantage for girls are apparent across the entire period, and can be seen to increase slightly in the older months before converging again at 30 months. However, because this accounts for a very small percentage of the variance, sex is a relatively minor contributor to individual variation in reported production vocabulary levels for children in this sample. The fitted percentile values for both sexes combined, girls, and boys are presented in Tables 5.19, 5.20, and 5.21.

How Children Use Words   The section labeled How Children Use Words contains five items that assess the extent to which children use words to refer

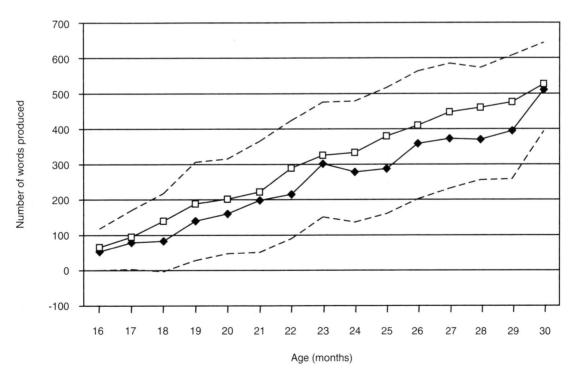

Figure 4.11.   Mean Words Produced (CDI: Words and Sentences) scores by age and sex. (*Note:* The dashed lines represent ±1 standard deviation for the sexes combined.) (*Key:* ◆ = boys; □ = girls.)

to the past or future or to missing or absent objects or people. *Sometimes* and *often* were combined to produce an affirmative category. Figure 4.12 shows the mean number of affirmative responses (5 possible) on this section by age, and Table 4.19 provides further descriptive information. The mean number of responses increased over the 16- to 30-month period, demonstrating a generally monotonic trend with age. Variation in scores was quite substantial, spanning the entire range of possible scores at almost each age. There is some suggestion that the variation tends to decrease in the later months.

The mean number of affirmative responses is presented for girls and boys separately at each age in Figure 4.13. Totals on this measure were analyzed with a 2 (sex) × 15 (age) between-subjects ANOVA. This analysis yielded significant main effects of age, $F(14, 1431) = 28.4$, $p < .0001$, and sex, $F(1, 1431) = 16.2$, $p < .0001$, as well as a significant age by sex interaction, $F(14, 1431) = 2.1$, $p < .02$. Age accounted for 22% of the variance, sex accounted for approximately 1% of the variance, and the age by sex interaction accounted for approximately 2% of the variance. Planned comparisons between girls and boys at each age indicated that sex differences were reliable only at 16, 18, and 19 months, $p < .05$. Thus, in addition to accounting for the small amount of variance, mean differences contributing to the significant main effect of sex are apparent only at early time points. This again suggests a relatively minor contribution of sex to the individual variation that is observed in this measure.

Differences in the developmental pace of acquisition for each of the 5 items in this section are displayed in Table 4.20. As can be seen, references to the past and future emerged later than references to absent owners and absent objects.

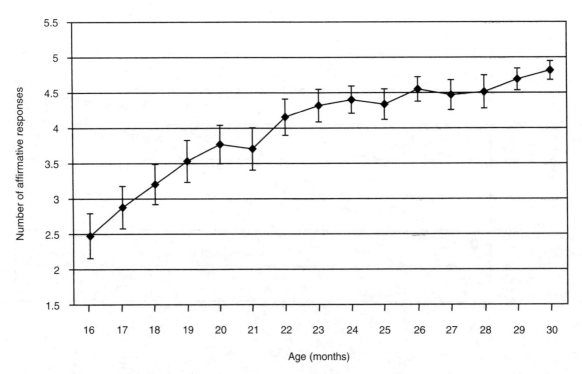

Figure 4.12. Mean How Children Use Words (CDI: Words and Sentences) scores by age in months. (*Note:* Bars above and below each mean score represent the 95% confidence intervals.)

Table 4.19. Descriptive statistics for How Children Use Words (CDI: Words and Sentences)

Age in months	n	M	Mdn	SD	Standard error of the mean	Minimum	Maximum[a]
16	74	2.5	2.0	1.4	0.2	0	5
17	81	2.9	3.0	1.4	0.2	0	5
18	103	3.2	3.0	1.5	0.1	0	5
19	98	3.5	4.0	1.5	0.1	0	5
20	117	3.8	4.0	1.5	0.1	0	5
21	95	3.7	4.0	1.5	0.2	0	5
22	90	4.2	5.0	1.2	0.1	1	5
23	104	4.3	5.0	1.2	0.1	0	5
24	135	4.4	5.0	1.1	0.1	0	5
25	107	4.3	5.0	1.1	0.1	0	5
26	100	4.5	5.0	0.9	0.1	0	5
27	113	4.5	5.0	1.1	0.1	0	5
28	84	4.5	5.0	1.1	0.1	0	5
29	80	4.7	5.0	0.7	0.1	2	5
30	80	4.8	5.0	0.6	0.1	2	5

[a]Maximum score possible = 5.

Key: n = number; *M* = mean; *Mdn* = median; *SD* = standard deviation.

A similar trend was found in the original normative sample of English-speaking toddlers (see Table 4.11 on p. 56 in Fenson et al., 1992/1993).

Word Endings/Part 1   The use of suffixes to designate plurals and other grammatical forms is a clear sign of linguistic growth. This ability is assessed in the section Word Endings/Part 1. As shown dramatically in Figure 4.14, the period from 16- to 30-months (for which the CDI: Words and Sentences is de-

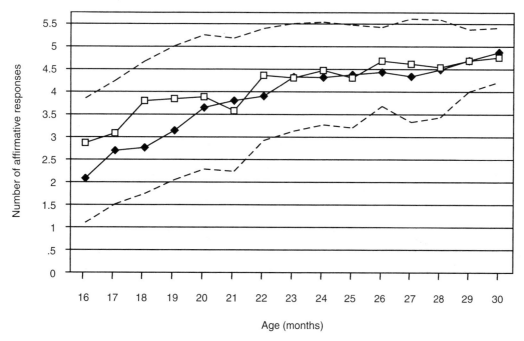

Figure 4.13.   Mean How Children Use Words (CDI: Words and Sentences) scores by age and sex. (*Note:* The dashed lines represent ±1 standard deviation for the sexes combined.) (*Key:* ◆ = boys; □ = girls.)

Table 4.20. Percentage of children with affirmative (*sometimes* or *often*) responses for items in How Children Use Words (CDI: Words and Sentences)

	How Children Use Words				
Age in months	Past	Future	Absent object (production)	Absent object (comprehension)	Absent owner
16	17.6	18.9	60.8	90.5	59.5
17	27.2	34.6	65.4	93.8	66.7
18	37.9	43.7	72.8	91.3	74.8
19	46.9	54.1	79.6	90.8	81.6
20	57.3	60.7	80.3	95.7	82.9
21	56.8	55.8	81.1	93.7	83.2
22	68.9	70.0	86.7	98.9	91.1
23	77.9	74.0	91.3	95.2	93.3
24	80.0	78.5	88.9	97.8	94.8
25	75.7	78.5	90.7	95.3	93.5
26	82.0	85.0	93.0	98.0	97.0
27	86.7	82.3	89.4	95.6	92.9
28	85.7	83.3	90.5	96.4	95.2
29	88.8	86.3	97.5	98.8	97.5
30	93.8	93.8	96.3	98.8	98.8

signed) almost perfectly brackets the developmental course of the four grammatical forms sampled, from preemergence to common use. At 16 months, the use of these forms is just beginning for most children. By 30 months, most children in the sample were reported to use all four of these morphological markers.

Differences in the rate of emergence of these four grammatical forms are illustrated in Table 4.21. Uses of the plural -*s*, the possessive -*s*, and the progres-

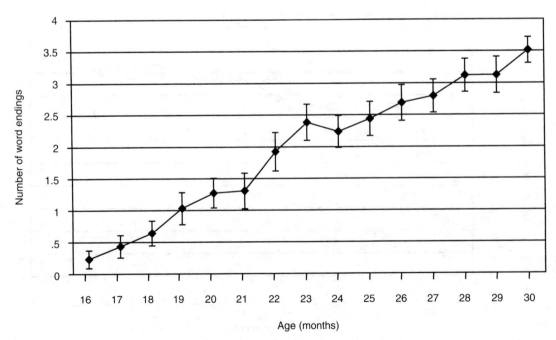

Figure 4.14. Mean Word Endings/Part 1 (CDI: Words and Sentences) scores by age in months. (*Note:* Bars above and below each mean score represent the 95% confidence intervals.)

Table 4.21. Percentage of children with affirmative (*sometimes* or *often*) responses for items in Word Endings/Part 1 (CDI: Words and Sentences)

Age in months	Word Endings/Part 1			
	Plural -*s*	Possessive -*s*	Progressive -*ing*	Past tense -*ed*
16	10.8	8.1	4.1	0
17	16.0	18.5	4.9	3.7
18	27.2	21.4	13.6	1.9
19	44.9	30.6	18.4	9.2
20	41.9	47.0	27.4	11.1
21	42.1	48.4	27.4	12.6
22	58.9	64.4	47.8	21.1
23	69.2	75.0	60.6	33.7
24	63.0	70.4	55.6	34.8
25	69.2	73.8	64.5	36.4
26	78.0	79.0	64.0	48.0
27	76.1	84.1	69.0	50.4
28	85.7	85.7	82.1	58.3
29	82.5	86.3	80.0	63.8
30	92.5	91.3	93.8	73.8

sive -*ing* morphemes were reported for at least a few of the children at 16 months, whereas, no 16-month-old children were reported to produce the past tense -*ed* suffix. The developmental lag in the past tense -*ed* morpheme is apparent throughout the period. At 24 months, more than half of the children were reported to produce plural -*s*, the possessive -*s*, and the progressive -*ing*, but only about one third of the children were reported to use the past tense form. By 30 months, nearly all of the children used the three early appearing forms (plural, possessive, progressive), but one quarter of the children still did not use the past tense form. These general patterns are quite similar to previous findings based on naturalistic language samples (e.g., Bates et al., 1988; Brown, 1973; deVilliers & deVilliers, 1973).

Word Forms　The acquisition of correct irregular word forms represents another clear sign of morphological progress. This ability is assessed in the Word Forms section of CDI: Words and Sentences. Figure 4.15 shows the average number of irregular forms (by age) checked by parents, and Table 4.22 presents more complete descriptive statistics for this measure. At 16 months, use of these forms was reported to be very infrequent (as it should be, based on the literature). Use of irregular words accelerated in the third year; by 30 months, a majority of children were reported to be producing about half of the nouns and verbs on the list. Fitted percentile tables for irregular nouns and verbs for both sexes combined, girls, and boys appear in Tables 5.22, 5.23, and 5.24.

Word Endings/Part 2　The overregularized nouns and verbs listed in the Word Endings/Part 2 section are "mistakes" from an adult point of view. However, psycholinguists view them as a sign of progress in acquiring linguistic rules and regularities (Berko, 1958; Brown, 1973; Bybee & Slobin, 1982; Marchman & Bates, 1994; Marcus et al., 1992). As shown in Table 4.23, use of these forms increases steadily across the age range. However, the number of these

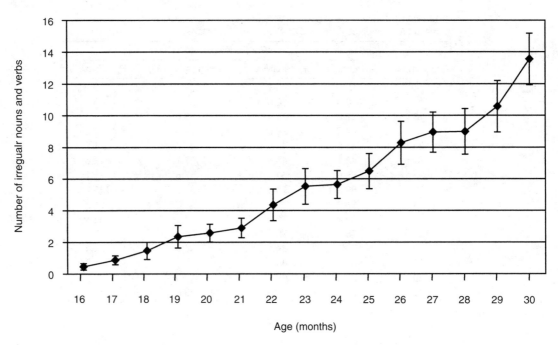

Figure 4.15. Mean Word Forms (CDI: Words and Sentences) scores by age in months. (*Note:* Bars above and below each mean score represent the 95% confidence intervals.)

forms reported to be in use remained relatively low, especially prior to the beginning of the child's third year of life. At the same time, there is considerable individual variation in the reported use of noun and verb overgeneralizations. At every age, at least a few children did not produce any of the overgeneralized forms, whereas at 25 and 27 months of age, at least one child produced almost all of them. Figure 4.16 shows the mean number of overgeneralized nouns and

Table 4.22. Descriptive statistics for Word Forms (CDI: Words and Sentences)

Age in months	n	M	Mdn	SD	Standard error of the mean	Minimum	Maximum[a]
16	74	0.5	.0	0.9	0.1	0	4
17	81	0.9	.0	1.3	0.1	0	6
18	103	1.5	1.0	2.8	0.3	0	23
19	98	2.3	1.0	3.6	0.4	0	24
20	117	2.6	2.0	3.1	0.3	0	17
21	95	2.9	2.0	3.1	0.3	0	15
22	90	4.4	3.0	4.7	0.5	0	22
23	104	5.5	4.0	5.7	0.6	0	23
24	135	5.6	4.0	5.1	0.4	0	25
25	107	6.5	4.0	5.8	0.6	0	25
26	100	8.3	6.0	6.8	0.7	0	25
27	113	8.9	7.0	6.8	0.6	0	25
28	84	9.0	8.0	6.6	0.7	0	25
29	80	10.6	10.0	7.3	0.8	0	25
30	80	13.6	13.0	7.3	0.8	1	25

[a]Maximum score possible = 25.

Key: n = number; *M* = mean; *Mdn* = median; *SD* = standard deviation.

Table 4.23.   Descriptive statistics for Word Endings/Part 2 (CDI: Words and Sentences)

Age in months	n	M	Mdn	SD	Standard error of the mean	Minimum	Maximum[a]
16	74	0.1	0.0	0.6	0.1	0	4
17	81	0.2	0.0	0.8	0.1	0	5
18	103	0.5	0.0	1.8	0.2	0	13
19	98	1.1	0.0	2.9	0.3	0	18
20	117	0.8	0.0	1.8	0.2	0	9
21	95	1.0	0.0	2.0	0.2	0	9
22	90	1.8	0.0	2.6	0.3	0	11
23	104	2.0	1.0	2.8	0.3	0	13
24	135	2.6	0.0	3.9	0.3	0	19
25	107	2.7	0.0	6.6	0.6	0	45
26	100	4.0	3.0	4.3	0.4	0	18
27	113	4.2	2.0	5.9	0.6	0	44
28	84	3.9	2.0	4.5	0.5	0	18
29	80	4.1	3.0	4.5	0.5	0	21
30	80	5.5	4.5	5.7	0.6	0	37

[a]Maximum score possible = 45.

Key: n = number; *M* = mean; *Mdn* = median; *SD* = standard deviation.

verbs reported to be in use at each month across the CDI: Words and Sentences age range.

Combining   The final portion of the CDI: Words and Sentences form focuses on the acquisition of word combinations and more complex syntactic forms. Parents were first asked whether their child had begun to combine words. The ability to combine words is a fundamental aspect of linguistic growth that

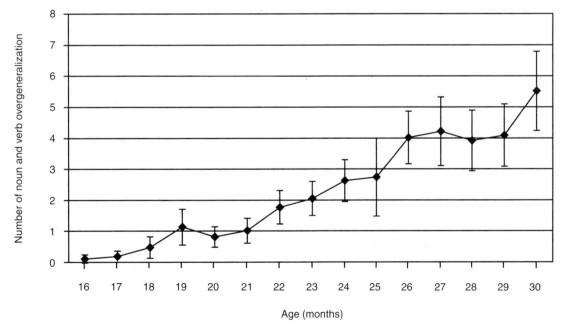

Figure 4.16.   Mean Word Endings/Part 2 (CDI: Words and Sentences) scores by age and sex. (*Note:* Bars above and below each mean score represent the 95% confidence intervals.)

sets the stage for a wide array of syntactic and semantic developments. Parents were given three options for responding: *not yet, sometimes,* and *often.* The *sometimes* category was included to obtain evidence of combining from parents who may be too conservative in their assessment, because even the presence of a few beginning combinations is potentially noteworthy (i.e., *sometimes* and *often* responses were grouped together as affirmative responses). Table 4.24 shows the remarkably regular progression in parents' responses to this question across the 16- to 30-month age period. Figure 4.17 presents the mean reported scores for this measure by age and sex. The percentage of children reported to be combining words rose steadily with age for both girls and boys. These results provide an excellent match to the results obtained in observational studies on the timing of first word combinations (Bates et al., 1988; Braine, 1976; Dromi, 1987).

Frequencies of combining were analyzed with a 2 (sex) × 15 (age) between-subjects ANOVA on the three-level response variable. This analysis yielded significant main effects of age, $F(14, 1429) = 31.4$, $p < .0001$, and sex, $F(1, 1429) = 12.9$, $p < .001$, as well as a significant age by sex interaction, $F(14, 1429) = 1.8$, $p < .03$. Age accounted for approximately 23.5% of the variance, sex accounted for 0.9% of the variance, and the age by sex interaction accounted for approximately 1.8% of the variance. Planned comparisons indicated significant gender effects only at the 18- and 19-month time points ($p < .05$).

Example Utterances   Parents who indicated that their children had begun to combine words were then asked, "Please list three of the longest sentences you have heard your child say recently." M3L was computed for each child following procedures adapted from Miller (1981) as described in the coding guidelines in the Chapter 2 heading called "Scoring the Child's Three Longest Sentences."

Table 4.24. Percentage of children with *not yet* and affirmative (*sometimes* or *often*) responses in Combining (CDI: Words and Sentences)

Age in months	Girls		Boys	
	not yet	*sometimes* or *often*	*not yet*	*sometimes* or *often*
16	64.9	35.1	78.4	21.6
17	50.0	50.0	67.4	32.6
18	34.1	65.9	55.9	44.1
19	21.8	78.2	46.5	53.5
20	30.0	70.0	31.6	68.4
21	27.5	72.5	27.3	72.7
22	14.0	86.0	27.5	72.5
23	15.4	84.6	3.9	96.1
24	14.1	85.9	14.3	85.7
25	1.7	98.3	12.5	87.5
26	4.3	95.7	11.3	88.7
27	3.7	96.3	8.5	91.5
28	2.4	97.6	4.7	95.3
29	2.6	97.4	0	100.0
30	0	100.0	0	100.0

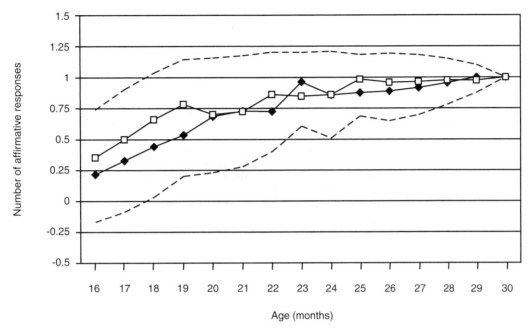

Figure 4.17. Mean Combining (CDI: Words and Sentences) scores by age and sex. (*Note:* The dashed lines represent ±1 standard deviation for the sexes combined.) (*Key:* ◆ = boys; □ = girls.)

M3L was computed by adding the number of morphemes in each utterance and dividing by the number of utterances provided. In a few cases, the parent indicated that the child had begun to combine words, but the parent did not offer any examples. In these cases, the score was reported as missing data. If the parent did not report that the child was combining words but provided examples of scorable multimorphemic utterances, the score for Combining was adjusted to indicate that the child was combining words. The same was done if the parent did not report that the child was combining words but selected the Complexity section. In each case, the scores for Examples/M3L and Complexity were summed and used.

Figure 4.18 presents the average Examples/M3L scores as a function of age. Sentence length increased rather steadily from about 1.5 morphemes at 16 months to 8 morphemes at 30 months. Note that the variation in range of scores is considerably smaller during the early months than the later ages due to the fact that at the earlier months the majority of the children in the sample were not yet reported to produce word combinations. Table 4.25 presents more complete descriptive statistics for Examples/M3L.

Figure 4.19 presents mean Examples/M3L scores for boys and girls in each age group. A 2 (sex) × 15 (age) between-subjects ANOVA for Examples/M3L yielded a significant main effect of sex, $F(1, 1381) = 29.9$, $p < .0001$, and a significant main effect of age, $F(14, 1381) = 54.2$, $p < .0001$. Age accounted for 35.5% of the variance, and sex accounted for approximately 2% of the variance. No significant age by sex interaction was found, $F(14, 1381) = 1.4$, *ns*. This finding suggests that the relatively minor effect of sex was relatively constant across the period here, although it might appear to be more evident in the later

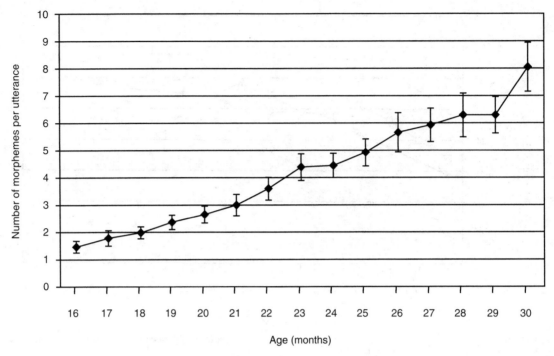

Figure 4.18. Examples/mean length of the three longest sentences (M3L) (CDI: Words and Sentences) scores by age in months. (*Note:* Bars above and below each mean score represent the 95% confidence intervals.)

months (see Figure 4.19). The percentiles for both sexes combined, girls, and boys are found in Tables 5.28, 5.29, and 5.30.

It should be kept in mind that although M3L is substantially correlated with mean length of utterance (MLU) based on a language sample (see Table 4.35 later in this chapter)—and thus is a valid measure of relative grammatical development—the actual values for M3L will generally be substantially higher than MLU. M3L should not be interpreted as an estimate of MLU.

Complexity   Each of the 37 sentence pairs in the Complexity section contains a more and a less complicated phrase or sentence expressing approximately the same meaning. The first sentence in each pair is the simpler version. The parent could select either or neither sentence. If the parent checked the less complex sentence in a given pair, or if the parent left that item blank, a score of 0 was assigned for that item; if the parent checked the more complex alternative on a given item, or both alternatives, a score of 1 was assigned. The Complexity score represents the number of times the parents selected the more complex example of the pair (37 maximum). For children who were not yet reported to be combining words, this measure was set to 0. Figure 4.20 presents mean grammatical complexity scores by age in months, and Table 4.26 provides an overview of the descriptive statistics for grammatical complexity. As would be expected, the number of more complex examples that were selected by the parents increased as the children increased in age from 16 to 30

Table 4.25. Descriptive statistics for Examples/M3L (CDI: Words and Sentences)

Age in months	n	M	Mdn	SD	Standard error of the mean	Minimum	Maximum
16	73	1.5	1.0	0.9	0.1	1.0	4.7
17	81	1.8	1.0	1.3	0.1	1.0	9.3
18	102	2.0	2.0	1.1	0.1	1.0	6.0
19	96	2.4	2.3	1.3	0.1	1.0	7.3
20	112	2.7	2.3	1.7	0.2	1.0	9.3
21	93	3.0	3.0	1.9	0.2	1.0	11.7
22	85	3.6	3.3	1.9	0.2	1.0	8.7
23	98	4.4	3.7	2.4	0.2	1.0	12.0
24	131	4.4	4.0	2.6	0.2	1.0	12.0
25	106	4.9	4.7	2.6	0.3	1.0	16.0
26	99	5.7	5.3	3.6	0.4	1.0	21.3
27	111	5.9	5.0	3.3	0.3	1.0	24.0
28	79	6.3	6.0	3.6	0.4	1.0	20.3
29	75	6.3	6.3	2.9	0.3	1.0	14.0
30	70	8.0	7.0	3.8	0.4	2.7	24.7

Key: M3L = mean length of three longest sentences; *n* = number; *M* = mean; *Mdn* = median; *SD* = standard deviation.

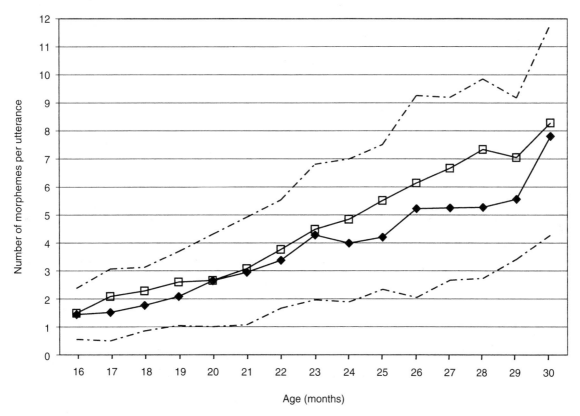

Figure 4.19. Examples/mean length of the three longest sentences (M3L) (CDI: Words and Sentences) scores by age and sex. (*Note:* The dashed lines represent ±1 standard deviation for the sexes combined.) (*Key:* ◆ = boys; □ = girls.)

months, with a somewhat more rapid trajectory after 25 months. In addition, there was considerably less variation in the scores at younger ages, when fewer children were reported to be producing any word combinations. These scores are similar to those observed in the original English norming study up to approximately 20 months of age. After this time, scores were slightly lower than those originally reported (see Figure 4.13 on p. 62 of Fenson et al., 1992/1993).

Examination of the "Minimum" and "Maximum" columns in Table 4.26 illustrates in still another way the wide variability in early language competencies. At every month, at least one child was reported to be using only the simpler forms. From 23 months on, one or more children at each age reached the maximum score of 37. Table 4.27 further illustrates this variability on the Complexity scale.

Mean scores for grammatical complexity for boys and girls at each age are shown in Figure 4.21. Results from a 2 (sex) × 15 (age) between-subjects ANOVA yielded a significant main effect of sex, $F(1, 1431) = 49.5$, $p < .001$, and a significant main effect of age, $F(14, 1431) = 65.7$, $p < .0001$. Age accounted for nearly 39% of the variance, whereas sex accounted for just slightly more than 3%. As shown in Figure 4.21, the gender effect for Complexity was more evident in the later months (after 22 months), as evidenced by a significant age by sex interaction, $F(14, 1431) = 2.6$, $p < .001$. Planned comparisons between sex at each age, however, indicated that the effect of sex was statistically reliable only at the 25-, 26-, 28-, and 29-month time points ($p < .05$). Again, these results indicate a relatively minor role for sex in expressive language development in this age range.

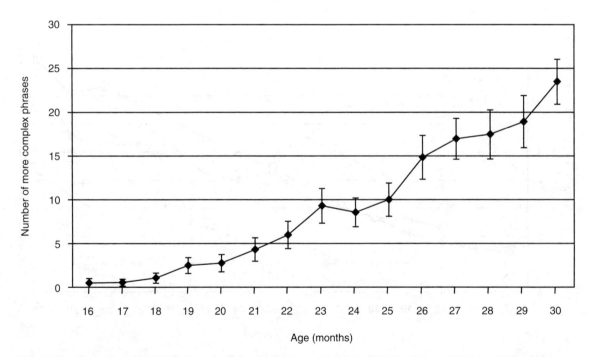

Figure 4.20.   Mean Complexity (CDI: Words and Sentences) scores by age in months. (*Note:* Bars above and below each mean score represent the 95% confidence intervals.)

Table 4.26. Descriptive statistics for Complexity (CDI: Words and Sentences)

Age in months	n	M	Mdn	SD	Standard error of the mean	Minimum	Maximum[a]
16	74	0.5	0.0	2.1	0.2	0	12
17	81	0.5	0.0	1.8	0.2	0	9
18	103	1.0	0.0	3.0	0.3	0	23
19	98	2.4	0.0	4.5	0.5	0	26
20	117	2.7	0.0	5.2	0.5	0	27
21	95	4.3	1.0	6.5	0.7	0	29
22	90	5.8	4.0	7.1	0.7	0	29
23	104	9.4	5.5	10.0	1.0	0	37
24	135	8.5	5.0	9.4	0.8	0	37
25	107	9.9	7.0	9.9	1.0	0	37
26	100	14.7	12.5	12.5	1.3	0	37
27	113	16.7	16.0	12.5	1.2	0	37
28	84	17.9	18.5	12.3	1.3	0	37
29	80	18.9	19.0	12.6	1.4	0	37
30	80	22.9	25.5	11.4	1.3	0	37

[a]Maximum score possible = 37.

Key: n = number; *M* = mean; *Mdn* = median; *SD* = standard deviation.

IMPACT OF DEMOGRAPHIC FACTORS ON LANGUAGE OUTCOMES

Maternal Education

Maternal education was adopted as an index of socioeconomic status (SES) for two reasons. First, it is more easily and reliably obtained than other indices of SES, such as family income. Second, it has traditionally been a strong correlate of other measures of SES and of direct measures of parental interaction with

Table 4.27. Percentage of children with Complexity (CDI: Words and Sentences) scores falling in four successive ranges

Age in months	Complexity scores			
	0	1–10	11–20	21–37[a]
16	91.9	5.4	2.7	0
17	87.7	12.3	0	0
18	78.6	19.4	1.0	1.0
19	52.0	40.8	6.1	1.0
20	58.1	36.8	1.7	3.4
21	44.2	41.1	10.5	4.2
22	34.4	46.7	11.1	7.8
23	16.3	50.0	19.2	14.4
24	23.7	44.4	17.0	14.8
25	15.0	47.7	22.4	15.0
26	15.0	30.0	20.0	35.0
27	9.7	27.4	22.1	40.7
28	10.7	21.4	20.2	47.6
29	10.0	20.0	23.8	46.3
30	2.5	18.8	16.3	62.5

[a]Maximum score possible = 37.

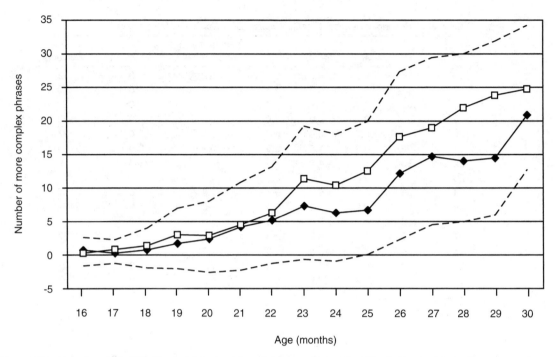

Figure 4.21. Mean Complexity (CDI: Words and Sentences) scores by age and sex. (*Note:* The dashed lines represent ±1 standard deviation for the sexes combined.) (*Key:* ◆ = boys; □ = girls.)

children (Dollaghan et al., 1999; Garcia Coll, 1990; Jackson-Maldonado, Thal, Marchman, Bates, & Gutierrez-Clellen, 1993; Laosa, 1984; Walker, Greenwood, Hart, & Carta, 1994). For the analyses described here, maternal education was divided into two levels: high school or less (i.e., 12 or fewer years of education) and more than high school (i.e., 13 or more years of education). The sample for CDI: Words and Gestures was divided into two age periods (8–12 months and 13–18 months). The CDI: Words and Sentences sample was divided into three age periods (16–20 months, 21–25 months, and 26–30 months). This grouping strategy ensured that there was a sufficient number of children at each age and education level. Multivariate analyses of variance (age level, education level) were conducted for four key CDI: Words and Gestures measures (Phrases Understood, Words Understood, Words Produced, and Total Gestures), and three key CDI: Words and Sentences measures (Words Produced, Examples/M3L, and Complexity).

Figure 4.22 presents the mean number of phrases understood (from CDI: Words and Gestures) as a function of age group and maternal education. Effects were evaluated using a 2 (age) × 2 (education) between-subjects ANOVA. This analysis indicated significant main effects of age group, $F(1, 1082) = 403.7, p < .0001$, and maternal education level, $F(1, 1082) = 5.3, p < .03$, as well as an age X education interaction, $F(1, 1082) = 10.5, p < .001$. Age accounted for approximately 27% of the variance, whereas maternal education accounted for approximately 0.5% of the variance. The interaction accounted for approximately 1% of the variance. Thus, as for sex, maternal education accounted for a very small amount of variance in early comprehension of phrases. Examination of Figure 4.22 indicates that mean scores for 8- to 12-month-old children whose mothers had less education (high school or less; $M = 13.8$, $SD = 6.4$) were higher than those of the children whose mothers had more education ($M = 11.5$, $SD = 6.4$, $p < .001$). However, the mean number of phrases understood did not differ based on maternal education at the older ages ($M = 20.7$, $SD = 6.1$; $M = 21.1$, $SD = 5.9$ for the high school or less and more than high school groups, respectively).

Figure 4.23 presents the mean number of words understood at each age for both levels of education. Effects were evaluated using a 2 (age group) × 2 (education) between-subjects ANOVA. This analysis revealed a main effect of age group, $F(1, 1082) = 427.1$, $p < .0001$. The interaction between age group and education approached significance, $F(1, 1082) = 3.8$, $p < .06$; however, the overall main effect of maternal education was not significant, $F(2, 1082) = 0.5$, ns. Age group accounted for approximately 28% of the variance, and the interaction accounted for less than 1% of the variance, indicating a very small effect of maternal education on vocabulary comprehension. Planned contrasts indicated that at 8–12 months of age, children whose mothers had less education had higher reported comprehension vocabularies ($M = 72.9$, $SD = 58.5$) than children whose mothers had some college ($M = 59.4$, $SD = 56.1$), $p < .02$. Yet, mean vocabulary comprehension scores did not differ as a function of maternal education at the older ages ($M = 169.8$ $SD = 99.7$ and $M = 176.3$, $SD = 93.1$ for the high school or less and more than high school groups, respectively).

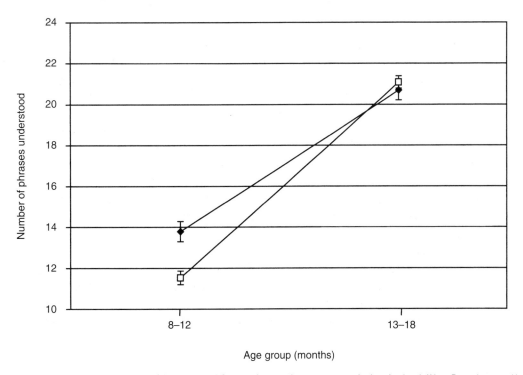

Figure 4.22. Mean Phrases Understood (CDI: Words and Gestures) scores by age group and education level. (*Note:* Bars above and below each mean score represent the standard error of the mean.) (*Key:* ◆ = high school or less; □ = more than high school.)

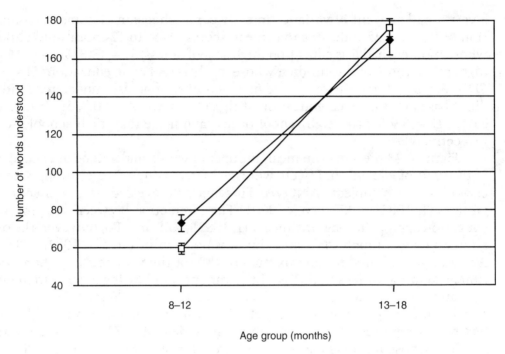

Figure 4.23. Mean Words Understood (CDI: Words and Gestures) scores by age group and education level. (*Note:* Bars above and below each mean score represent the standard error of the mean.) (*Key:* ◆ = high school or less; □ = more than high school.)

These findings closely parallel the results of the original English CDI norming study, in which significantly higher scores for vocabulary comprehension at the youngest ages were reported for children of mothers with lower education than for children of mothers with higher education (Fenson et al., 1992/1993). Parallel results were obtained in the Mexican Spanish CDIs normative study (Jackson-Maldonado et al., 2003). The findings are also consistent with an earlier report by Reznick (1990), in which he noted that parents with lower education gave higher estimates of vocabulary comprehension for their 12-month-old sons than did parents with higher educational backgrounds. More recently, Feldman et al. (2000) reported a similar, inverse relation between education level and scores on three measures from the CDI: Words and Gestures form (Phrases Understood, Words Understood, and Words Produced), also limited to the 8- to 12-month age range. It is possible that children of mothers with less education have higher comprehension vocabularies, but this hypothesis does not seem plausible. An alternative explanation is that these mothers are less objective in their interpretation of their infants' comprehension vocabulary, either exaggerating the infants' knowledge or failing to be appropriately cautious in judgments of what their children know. Because of these findings, the word comprehension measure for children younger than 1 year of age should be treated with caution, particularly with children whose parents have lower education levels.

The mean number of words produced on the CDI: Words and Gestures form for both education levels are shown in Figure 4.24. A 2 (age) × 2 (education) between-subjects ANOVA for vocabulary production revealed a significant main effect of age group, $F(1, 1082) = 188.8$, $p < .0001$, but no main effect of maternal education, $F(1, 1082) = 0.01$, *ns*, and no interaction $F(1, 1082) = 0.42$, *ns*. Age accounted for approximately 15% of the variance. Thus, unlike the previously reported comprehension measures, level of maternal education did not appear to influence the scores for words produced. A parallel result was obtained in the Mexican Spanish normative study.

The mean number of all gestures reported (Total Gestures Score) as a function of education and age group is shown in Figure 4.25. Results of a 2 (age group) × 2 (education level) between-subjects ANOVA indicated a significant main effect of age group, $F(1, 1075) = 782.6$, $p < .001$, and a significant age group by education level interaction, $F(1, 1075) = 12.0$, $p < .001$. There was no main effect of maternal education level, $F(1, 1075) = 0.3$, *ns*. Planned comparisons indicated that at 8–12 months of age, mothers in the least educated group reported more gestures ($M = 21.2$, $SD = 9.3$) compared with mothers in the more educated group ($M = 18.7$, $SD = 9.9$), $p < .01$. However, in the 13- to 18-month period, mothers who had less education were likely to report fewer gestures ($M = 37.6$, $SD = 11.3$) compared with mothers who had more education ($M = 39.8$, $SD = 10.3$), $p < .03$. These results are similar to those reported previously in the chapter regarding vocabulary comprehension for the present data and for the Mexican Spanish normative data.

Figure 4.26 presents the mean Words Produced scores on CDI: Words and Sentences as a function of age and education level. Results of a 3 (age group) × 2 (education) between-subjects ANOVA revealed a significant main effect of age

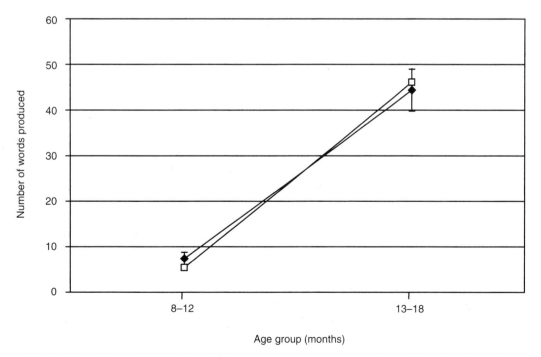

Figure 4.24. Mean Words Produced (CDI: Words and Gestures) scores by age group and education level. (*Note:* Bars above and below each mean score represent the standard error of the mean.) (*Key:* ◆ = high school or less; □ = more than high school.)

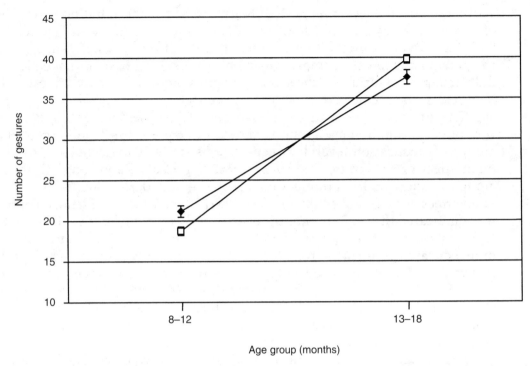

Figure 4.25. Mean Total Gestures (CDI: Words and Gestures) scores by age group and education level. (*Note:* Bars above and below each mean score represent the standard error of the mean.) (*Key:* ◆ = high school or less; □ = more than high school.)

group, $F(2, 1454) = 343.2$, $p < .0001$, a significant main effect of maternal education, $F(1, 1454) = 9.4$, $p < .002$, and a significant age group by education interaction, $F(2, 1454) = 5.1$, $p < .006$. Age group accounted for 32% of the variance, maternal education accounted for 0.6% of the variance, and the interaction accounted for 0.7% of the variance. Planned comparisons at each of the three levels of age indicated that mothers in the more educated group reported that their children produced a significantly greater number of words on average than the mothers with only high school or less education at the 21–25 month ($M = 300.1$, $SD = 171.2$ versus $M = 264.3$, $SD = 175.1$) and 26–30 month ($M = 448.1$, $SD = 166.6$ versus $M = 390.6$, $SD = 173.7$) groups ($p < .05$). Scores for the two education levels in the 16–20 month group were not significantly different.

Mean scores for Examples/M3L at the two education levels are shown in Figure 4.27. Results of a 3 (age group) × 2 (education) between-subjects ANOVA revealed a significant main effect of age group, $F(2, 1404) = 247.5$, $p < .0001$, a significant main effect of education, $F(2, 1404) = 30.3$, $p < .001$, and a significant age group by education interaction, $F(2, 1404) = 10.9$, $p < .001$. Age group accounted for 26% of the variance, education level accounted for 2% of the variance, and the interaction accounted for 1.5% of the variance. Planned comparisons indicated no significant differences based on level of maternal education at the earliest age group (16–20 months). Significant group differences, however, were found at 21–25 and 26–30 months of age ($p < .05$). In the 21–25 age group, the mean Examples/M3L score for the highest education group ($M = 4.5$,

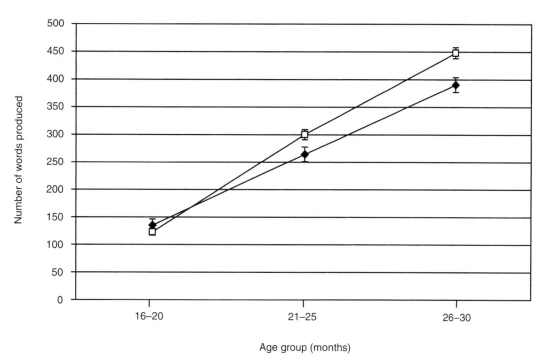

Figure 4.26. Mean Words Produced (CDI: Words and Sentences) scores by age group and education level. (*Note:* Bars above and below each mean score represent the standard error of the mean.) (*Key:* ◆ = high school or less; □ = more than high school.)

$SD = 2.6$) was significantly higher than that for the high school or less group ($M = 3.4$, $SD = 1.9$). Similarly, in the 26–30 month age group, the mean score was significantly higher in the more than high school education group ($M = 6.9$, $SD = 3.8$) than in the high school of less group ($M = 5.4$, $SD = 2.8$).

Figure 4.28 illustrates the differences in Complexity by age and education level. A 3 (age group) × 2 (education) between-subjects ANOVA revealed a significant main effect of age group, $F(2, 1454) = 312.3$, $p < .0001$, a significant main effect of maternal education, $F(1, 1454) = 14.7$, $p < .0001$, and a significant age by education interaction, $F(2, 1454) = 7.2$, $p < .001$. Age accounted for approximately 30% of the variance, education level accounted for 1% of the variance, and the interaction accounted for 1% of the variance. As was the case for Examples/M3L, no significant differences in Complexity scores were found for children with mothers from the two levels of education at 16–20 months. At 21–25 months and 26–30 months, however, analyses indicated that mean Complexity scores were significantly higher for children whose mothers were the most educated (21–25 months: $M = 6.9$, $SD = 3.7$; 26–30 months: $M = 19.6$, $SD = 12.5$) compared with children whose mothers had lower levels of education (21–25 months: $M = 5.4$, $SD = 2.8$; 26–30 months: $M = 15.2$, $SD = 12.1$), $p < .05$. Thus, the more familiar positive relation between SES and language skills was found for the three main CDI: Words and Sentences measures (Vocabulary Production, Examples/M3L, and Complexity); for each scale, this effect was statistically reliable only for the older two age groups (21–25 months

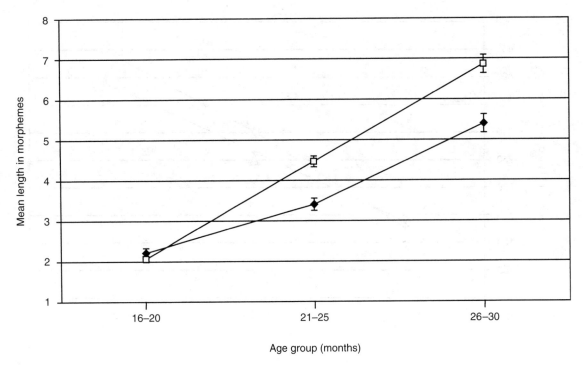

Figure 4.27. Examples/mean length of the three longest sentences (M3L) (CDI: Words and Sentences) scores by age group and education level. (*Note:* Bars above and below each mean score represent the standard error of the mean.) (*Key:* ◆ = high school or less; □ = more than high school.)

and 26–30 months). As for all of the other measures, however, maternal education accounted for only a very small amount of the variance in development of this aspect of language, suggesting that it is of relatively low practical significance, at least across the range of maternal education represented in the norming sample (approximately 93% of whom had a high school diploma or more).

Although the present norming sample is strongly skewed toward middle- and upper–middle-class children, the sample was sufficiently diverse to permit a reasonable assessment of the effects of socioeconomic status of the distribution of scores in both the CDI: Words and Gestures and the CDI: Words and Sentences data sets. The results of these assessments, together with the findings of related studies discussed in Chapter 2 (see the section called "Using the Norms with Children from Families of Low Socioeconomic Status"), demonstrate several age-related patterns concerning the effect of maternal education on CDI measures.

First, for younger children in the age range of the CDI: Words and Gestures form, reported comprehension measures (Phrases Understood and Words Understood) were higher in children whose mothers had less education. The opposite pattern was seen for vocabulary and grammar production in reports of older children in the range of the CDI: Words and Sentences. In the latter cases, reported scores for vocabulary and grammar were higher for children with more highly educated mothers than they were those for children whose mothers had fewer years of education.

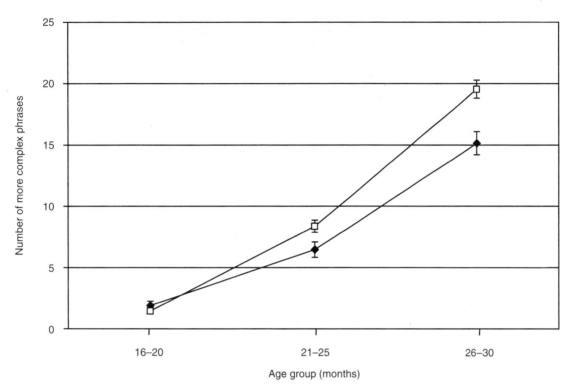

Figure 4.28.   Mean Complexity (CDI: Words and Sentences) scores by age group and education level. (*Note:* Bars above and below each mean score represent the standard error of the mean.) (*Key:* ◆ = high school or less; □ = more than high school.)

Despite the patterns found in the norming data, the small magnitude of these effects of maternal education on language development suggests that clinicians may feel comfortable using the CDI scores in determining classifications of typically developing or delayed language in children from low SES backgrounds. Although caution should always be exercised in interpreting parent report information provided in such instances, the evidence to date suggests that CDI profiles can provide useful information about the language skills of this sector of the population. Nonetheless, special caution should be exercised in interpreting the CDI subscales for children between 8 and 12 months of age, as some parents with low education levels seem to overestimate or overreport their child's linguistic abilities. It should also be kept in mind that some low SES parents may underreport their children's language skills on the CDI: Words and Sentences form, although not all CDI-based studies have observed this outcome (e.g., Rodrique, 2001).

More systematic analyses of the relation between education level and the assessment of language outcome with parent report are necessary to more fully understand the bases of these effects and their implications for assessment. Among the questions to be addressed is the extent to which variations in the effects of parental education reflect the genuine capabilities of the child and how much they reflect reporting styles and competence of the parent.

We also need to learn more about the applicability of the CDIs with children from very low SES families (i.e., families in which the mother has less than a high school education). At present, we believe that use of the CDIs—especially in combination with other measures of language development—is well justified for children from families in which the mother has a high school diploma. Greater caution is urged when a CDI is completed by a parent with less than a high school education. In such instances, and indeed in all applications, an ideal assessment package will never be limited solely to parent report or any other single measures strategy.

Birth Order

Birth order effects on communicative development were evaluated for four measures for the CDI: Words and Gestures form (Phrases Understood, Words Understood, Words Produced, and Total Gestures) and three measures for the CDI: Words and Sentences form (Words Produced, Examples/M3L, and Complexity).

For the CDI: Words and Gestures form, analyses were conducted using a 2 (first born versus later born) $\times$ 2 (age group: 8–12 versus 13–18 months) ANOVA. The means are presented in Table 4.28. For the mean number of phrases understood, the results indicated that only the main effect of age was significant, $F(1,1059) = 530.3$, $p < .0001$, with no main effect of birth order or interaction of birth order with age group. For words understood, the only significant effect was age, $F(1,1059) = 531.1$, $p < .0001$. For the number of words produced, the results indicated a significant effect of age, $F(1,1059) = 228.8$, $p < .001$; a significant effect of birth order, $F(1,1059) = 16.5$, $p < .001$; and a significant age group by birth order interaction, $F(1,1059) = 10.3$, $p < .001$. These findings show that the effect of birth order was more prominent in the older age groups (first born: $M = 55.2$; later born: $M = 36.2$) than in the younger age groups (first born: $M = 7.1$; later born: $M = 4.9$). Estimates of the η_p^2, however, indicated that age accounted for 17.8% of the variance, whereas birth order accounted for 1.5% of the variance and the interaction accounted for approximately 1% of the variance. Thus, the effect of birth order on word production accounts for a relatively small portion of the variance in word production in this age range. Finally, for the total number of gestures produced, there was a main effect of age group, $F(1,1059) = 987.7$, $p < .001$, and a main effect of birth order, $F(1,1059) =$

Table 4.28. Means and standard deviations for key CDI: Words and Gestures variables by birth order

CDI: Words and Gestures variable	8–12 months		13–18 months	
	First born (n = 263)	Later born (n = 263)	First born (n = 271)	Later born (n = 266)
Phrases Understood	12.2	12.2	20.9	21.0
Words Understood	65.2	62.3	182.0	167.4
Words Produced	7.2	4.9	55.2	36.2
Total Gestures	20.5	18.6	39.5	38.8

Note: Later-born range = 2nd to 7th child in family.

Key: n = number.

4.7, p < .04, but no age group by birth order group interaction. Again, the significance of the birth order effect was substantially smaller ($\eta_p^2 = .004$) than the overall impact of the age ($\eta_p^2 = .48$).

For the CDI: Words and Sentences variables, we examined the effects of birth order (first born versus later born) in three age groups (16–20, 21–25, and 26–30 months) in a 2 (birth order) × 3 (age group) ANOVA. The means are presented in Table 4.29. There were significant effects of both age and birth order for all three measures, such that first-born children had higher scores than later-born children. For the two measures of grammar, there were significant birth order by age group interactions (M3L, $F[2,1400] = 9.5$, $p < .001$; Complexity: $F[2, 1450] = 14.3$, $p < .0001$). In both cases, the impact of birth order was more evident in the older age groups than in the younger age groups. Examination of the practical significance of these effects (η_p^2) indicated that birth order accounted for relatively little variance (2.5%–3.8%) in these measures, far less than the variance accounted for by age (32%–38%).

RELATIONS AMONG THE INVENTORY SUBSCALES

How highly associated are the various aspects of communication assessed by the Inventories? That is, to what extent should children be expected to score at comparable percentile levels on the various components of each inventory? Would it be unusual for a child to receive a percentile score of 85 on one component (e.g., Words Produced) and a percentile score of 40 or 35 or even lower on another component (e.g., Complexity)? In this section, the interrelations among the major components of each inventory are reported. Overall, the intercorrelations are moderate to high. Nonetheless, as shown throughout the section, considerable unevenness in the profiles of individual children is not uncommon.

Intercorrelations Among the Components of the CDI: Words and Gestures

Table 4.30 shows the intercorrelations among raw scores on the major components of the CDI: Words and Gestures. One particularly clear pattern that emerged is that gestures are more closely associated with vocabulary comprehension (single words and phrases) than with vocabulary production. Similar

Table 4.29. Descriptive statistics for key CDI: Words and Sentences variables as a function of age group and birth order

CDI: Words and Sentences variable	16–20 months		21–25 months		26–30 months	
	First born (n = 237)	Later born (n = 236)	First born (n = 247)	Later born (n = 283)	First born (n = 213)	Later born (n = 240)
Words Produced	144.1	109.3	320.9	260.4	471.7	389.3
M3L	2.3	1.9	4.6	3.7	7.3	5.5
Complexity	1.9	1.2	8.5	7.1	21.4	15.0

Note: Later-born range = 2nd to 8th child in family.

Key: n = number; M3L = mean length of the three longest sentences.

Table 4.30. Intercorrelations among the major components of CDI: Words and Gestures

CDI: Words and Gestures component	Words Understood	Words Produced	Total Gestures
Phrases Understood	.80/.65	.50/.25	.77/.55
Words Understood		.70/.55	.79/.58
Words Produced			.59/.34

Note: For all values in this table, *p* (probability) < .01 or better. The second value in each pair is the correlation with age partialled out.

patterns have been reported by Bates et al. (1989); Thal and Bates (1988); Tamis-LeMonda and Bornstein (1990); and Bates, Dale, and Thal (1995). In addition, the two comprehension measures (Phrases Understood and Words Understood) are more highly correlated with each other than either one is with vocabulary production (i.e., Words Produced). The correlation, however, between vocabulary comprehension and production is moderate, whereas that between phrases understood and vocabulary production is considerably lower.

Overall, these intercorrelations indicate that the major features of early communication assessed on the CDI: Words and Gestures are associated. Children who display more gestures at an earlier age than their peers can also be expected to understand more words than their peers and are likely to be using more words than average as well. Nonetheless, correlations of the magnitude seen in Table 4.30 allow for a great deal of variation in the profiles of individual children. This point is illustrated in Table 4.31, which displays the raw scores and percentile scores for the major CDI: Words and Gestures measures for 23 children drawn from the normative data set. Individual profiles for these children differ dramatically, some showing close correspondence among the various components, others showing varying degrees of dissociability among the scales. For example, Child #1 and Child #9 are at the very top of the distribution on each of the three measures. Child #19 is consistently at the lower end of the distribution. Child #20 scored near the middle of the distribution on each major component. In contrast, Child #2 scored high on comprehension and gestures and was average on production. Child #3 was high on vocabulary comprehension and low on vocabulary production and on gestures. Child #5 displayed a fairly common profile, scoring low on vocabulary production but well above average on vocabulary comprehension and on gestures. The other profiles shown in Table 4.31 illustrate some of the other patterns found in the sample.

As discussed in Chapter 2, in evaluating the degree of association or dissociation among a child's percentile scores, the absolute value of the scores should be taken into account. For example, in Table 4.31, when looking only at the percentile scores, Child #21 shows a high degree of similarity across the three scales. However, his 40% rank for production is based on only one reported word in his expressive vocabulary and may therefore be the product of a floor effect. Many children are just beginning the venture into productive vocabulary at this age. For such children, it is too early to make judgments about their expressive skills. The same can be said about Child #22, who also shows an impressive degree of consistency across the three scales. His age–score com-

Table 4.31. Selected individual profiles for CDI: Words and Gestures

Child	Age (in months)	Sex	Words Understood		Words Produced		Total Gestures	
			Score	%	Score	%	Score	%
#1	12	male	175	90	29	93	40	93
#2	14	male	219	87	16	63	45	90
#3	14	female	203	73	0	5	25	19
#4	16	female	260	69	6	11	33	15
#5	14	female	217	77	3	25	41	70
#6	11	male	44	46	13	88	29	83
#7	13	male	0	<1	0	15	18	15
#8	10	female	11	10	4	60	9	15
#9	11	female	396	99	213	99	41	96
#10	15	female	302	89	84	85	44	65
#11	13	male	52	26	1	25	37	82
#12	13	male	194	88	5	55	41	89
#13	14	male	243	91	7	44	33	55
#14	14	female	33	6	24	60	30	30
#15	11	male	11	9	2	57	13	20
#16	12	male	7	<1	0	25	0	<1
#17	14	female	203	73	0	5	25	19
#18	15	female	275	83	6	15	45	70
#19	17	male	9	<1	5	10	26	<1
#20	10	female	34	40	2	45	18	50
#21	12	male	59	41	1	40	20	35
#22	10	male	74	76	3	65	21	70
#23	8	female	1	<1	1	60	0	<1

bination for vocabulary production puts him at the 65th percentile based on the use of only three words and is not likely to be a reliable indicator of his subsequent rank. Child #23 shows a different extreme pattern, also based on a floor effect. Being credited with a single word earns this child a percentile score of 60, which dramatically contrasts with percentile scores of <1 for the other 2 measures. Obviously, it is far too early to make any meaningful judgments about the language skills of this child, except to say that she has not yet begun to show the skills tapped by the inventory.

Strong dissociations may also be found in children at ages where the range in the raw scores is not a contributing factor. Examples include Child #17, who ranks well above the median in vocabulary comprehension but very low on the other two measures. Child #11 ranks high on the gestures scale but low on the other two measures.

Intercorrelations Among the Components of the CDI: Words and Sentences

Table 4.32 shows the intercorrelations among the main components of the CDI: Words and Sentences form. The components of this form are moderately to strongly related, with vocabulary production (Words Produced) highly corre-

Table 4.32. Intercorrelations among the major components of CDI: Words and Sentences

CDI: Words and Sentences component	M3L	Complexity	Word Forms
Words Produced	.78/.64	.82/.72	.83/.75
M3L		.82/.72	.71/.57
Complexity			.83/.74

Note: For all values in this table, *p* (probability) < .01 or better. The second value in each pair is the correlation with age partialled out.
Key: M3L = mean length of the three longest sentences.

lated with two of the grammar scales (Examples/M3L and Complexity). Similar strong relations between the vocabulary and grammar sections of the CDI: Words and Sentences have been reported elsewhere (e.g., Bates & Goodman, 1999). Similar relations between vocabulary size and the onset of grammar are also evident using direct observation (e.g., Bates et al., 1988; Bates, Dale, & Thal, 1995; Dale et al., 2000; Marchman et al., 2004). These intercorrelations between vocabulary and grammar have played an important role in recent theoretical claims regarding the nature of language learning mechanisms—in particular, the degree to which vocabulary and grammar share computational resources and properties (Dale et al., 2000; Marchman, Martínez-Sussmann, & Dale, 2004).

Table 4.33 lists the raw scores and percentile scores on the CDI: Words and Sentences for a sample of 24 toddlers. Paralleling the infant data shown in Table 4.31, Table 4.33 shows considerable variation in the similarity of percentile levels for individual children. Some children rank at similar levels on each of the four measures (e.g., Child #1, Child #2, Child #5, Child #9). Other children are consistent except for one of the measures (e.g., Child #6, Child #8, Child #10, Child #15, Child #23). Some children show more mixed patterns of dissociation (e.g., Child #17, Child #18, Child #23). As with the CDI: Words and Gestures data, in many cases at the lower age range of the instrument, discrepant patterns are at least partly attributable to floor effects (e.g., Child #3, Child #4, Child #10, Child #12, Child #14). For example, because some skills are just beginning to emerge in the 16- to 20-month-range, Child #14 places at the 85th percentile for sentence complexity even though she is not yet combining words. (The reader is reminded that Chapter 2's "Additional Considerations" section strongly recommends caution at the beginning levels of each scale.)

As discussed in the Chapter 3 section "Clinical Applications of the Inventories," extreme variations sometimes have clinical implications. However, authentic dissociations (those not attributable to floor effects) are also relatively common in typically developing children. The meaning of these dissociations is a matter of substantial interest among both clinicians and researchers. The inventories should help us understand this phenomenon by facilitating cross-

Table 4.33. Selected individual profiles for CDI: Words and Sentences

Child	Age (in months)	Sex	Words Produced		Complexity		Word Forms		M3L	
			Score	%	Score	%	Score	%	Score	%
#1	27	male	118	10	0	15	0	5	2.3	14
#2	27	female	585	79	29	70	14	75	9.0	81
#3	17	female	10	6	0	75	0	65	1.0	25
#4	17	female	29	20	0	75	0	65	1.0	25
#5	30	female	373	18	5	13	4	10	2.7	<1
#6	20	male	345	91	3	89	0	45	6.0	96
#7	26	male	40	<1	2	35	0	5	3.0	29
#8	27	male	632	94	30	85	7	40	10.3	92
#9	29	male	656	94	35	90	23	90	11.0	90
#10	18	male	34	28	0	85	1	65	2.0	67
#11	20	male	211	73	1	85	3	75	3.3	79
#12	20	male	66	33	0	70	1	65	3.0	75
#13	17	female	14	9	0	75	0	65	1.0	25
#14	17	male	7	6	0	85	0	65	1.0	30
#15	29	male	536	66	30	68	9	25	10.0	85
#16	20	male	481	98	25	99	13	97	9.3	99
#17	28	male	298	28	33	85	5	23	4.3	35
#18	21	male	80	32	7	90	2	65	4.3	84
#19	17	female	46	32	0	75	1	75	1.0	25
#20	24	female	275	39	15	75	5	65	5.0	63
#21	21	female	192	48	0	50	1	50	1.0	<1
#22	24	male	478	86	10	82	3	50	7.5	91
#23	29	female	653	92	26	37	11	35	8.7	64
#24	30	female	622	69	24	27	17	60	10.7	75

Key: M3L = mean length of the three longest sentences.

sectional and longitudinal study of children with uneven profiles in early communicative skills.

RELIABILITY OF THE INVENTORIES

Reliability refers to the consistency with which the items on a test or scale yield comparable indices of the abilities being assessed. Three types of reliability are commonly used for evaluation of assessment instruments: internal consistency, test–retest reliability and inter-rater (or inter-tester) reliability (see Sattler, 1988). Estimation and interpretation of these measures of reliability for a parent-report measure present some particular difficulties. For example, artificially high reliability scores may result from a halo effect (i.e., parents who overestimate their child's language skills in all areas) or from a tendency for parents to remember and repeat previous estimates of their child's vocabulary regardless of their accuracy of these estimates. Inter-rater reliability is often impossible to estimate in the context of child language because there may be only one individual who is sufficiently familiar with the child's language abilities to be able to provide data. Consequently, although the internal consistency and test–retest analyses summarized in the following sections show generally impressive results, the best evidence for the reliability of the present measures comes from their substantial concurrent validity, as documented in the following section. This inference is justified by the conclusion from statistical theory (Lyman, 1998) that validity can never exceed reliability.

Internal Consistency

Internal consistency refers to the extent to which different items within the same category measure the same content domain. Internal consistency was evaluated by computing Cronbach's coefficient alpha. This index, based on the intercorrelations among all the items within a given category, yields what is essentially the average split-half correlation across all possible splits. Cronbach's alpha was computed for three scales on the CDI: Words and Gestures (Words Understood, Words Produced, Total Gestures) as well as for Words Produced and Complexity on the CDI: Words and Sentences form.

For each vocabulary measure, scores for each category were treated as individual items (there are 19 semantic categories on the CDI: Words and Gestures Vocabulary Checklist and 22 on the CDI: Words and Sentences Vocabulary Checklist, and there are 5 gesture categories on the CDI: Words and Gestures form). Coefficient alpha is an appropriate index to apply in this instance, given the relatively large number of categories and the conceptual coherence of the items making up each category.

The three vocabulary scales demonstrated high internal consistency— producing alpha values of .95, .96, and .96—for CDI: Words and Gestures Words Understood, CDI: Words and Gestures Words Produced, and CDI: Words and Sentences Words Produced, respectively. For CDI: Words and Gestures Words Understood and Words Produced measures, the only categories with corrected item–whole correlations below .70 were Words About Time (.65 for both) and Question Words (.68 and .56, respectively), reflecting their relatively low occurrence in this age range. For the CDI: Words and Sentences Words Produced measure, the categories with corrected item–whole correlations below .70 were Sound Effects and Animal Sounds (.65, a ceiling effect) and Connecting Words (.68).

On the CDI: Words and Gestures Gesture scale, Total Gestures demonstrated somewhat lower internal consistency, with an alpha coefficient of .88. Analysis of the intercorrelations revealed that two of the five subscales, Actions with Objects (Section C) and Imitating Other Adult Actions (Section E), were correlated above .85 with each other. The remaining three categories—First Communicative Gestures (Section A), Games and Routines (Section B), and Pretending to Be a Parent (Section D)—all correlated below .76. These results may reflect the separability of the various gesture categories with respect to their time of emergence as well as their nature.

The CDI: Words and Sentences Complexity scale was analyzed using the three subcategories: bound morphemes (items 1–12), functor words (items

13–24), and complex sentences (items 25–37). These three subscales demonstrated high internal consistency, with an alpha coefficient of .95 and corrected item–whole correlations above .86 in each case.

These measures of internal consistency indicate a very high degree of reliability for the major components of each inventory, with the possible exception of Total Gestures of the CDI: Words and Gestures Gesture scale; this scale appears to be a combination of two somewhat separable scales, each with good internal consistency.

Test–Retest Reliability

Test–retest reliability measures the extent to which scores remain stable across two or more test sessions. Given the rapidity with which language skills can change over short periods of time and the uneven rates of language development among children, one would not expect the rank order for a group of children to remain constant for an extended period of time, but a considerable degree of stability would certainly be expected over a period of 2 months or less. (Correlations across longer intervals are discussed later in this chapter, in the section called "Predictive Validity.") Short-term test–retest reliability was assessed at the New Haven site by sending families a second CDI shortly after they had returned their first CDI form. For CDI: Words and Sentences, 137 pairs of forms were available, with an average test–retest lag of 1.35 months (range: 0.9–2.37 months). The Pearson correlation values (r) between the test and retest scores were computed separately for each month. Stability was uniformly strong across time for vocabulary comprehension, with correlations in the upper .80s; the sole exception occurred for children assessed initially at 12 months, for whom the test–retest correlation dropped to .61 ($p < .01$). The lower reliability at 12 months is consistent with previous reports of a general cognitive reorganization that occurs at approximately 12 months (McCall, Eichorn, & Hogarty, 1977). Stability for production was low in the 8- to 10-month range, probably due to the restricted range (i.e., a floor effect), but stabilized in subsequent months, with correlations in the mid-.80s. Gesture scores were also in the .80 range for each monthly level on the CDI: Words and Gestures form except at 12 months, at which point a coefficient of .60 was obtained—parallel to the reduction in month-to-month stability for vocabulary comprehension (Words Understood).

For CDI: Words and Sentences, 216 pairs of tests were available, with an average test–retest lag of 1.38 months (range: 0.73–2.94 months). The test–retest correlation for vocabulary production was .95 ($p < .01$), with correlations above .90 at each age. Taken together, the test–retest data provide additional evidence of high reliability for the inventories.

Standard Error of Measurement   The standard error of measurement (SEM) is useful for interpreting individual scores. It should not be confused with the standard error of the mean, (discussed previously in the chapter regarding the descriptive statistics tables), which is useful for evaluating and comparing samples. The value of SEM may be estimated as

$$SEM = SD \times \sqrt{(1\text{-reliability})}$$

for which reliability may be conservatively estimated as .80 for the three main CDI: Words and Gestures measures and .90 for the two main CDI: Words and Sentences measures and for which the SD at each month for the appropriate measure can be found in Tables 4.10, 4.12, 4.14, 4.17, and 4.26.

A confidence interval may then be obtained around an individual score with the formula

obtained score $\pm$ z $\times$ SEM or
obtained score $\pm$ z $\times$ SD * .447 for CDI: Words and Gestures measures
obtained score $\pm$ z $\times$ SD * .316 for CDI: Words and Sentences measures

where z is determined by the degree of confidence desired. For the 90% confidence interval, z = 1.65; for the 95% confidence interval, z = 1.96; and for the 99% confidence interval, z = 2.58. These calculations permit the evaluation of differences between scores on separate scales; if the confidence intervals determined in this fashion for the two scores do not overlap, the difference is statistically significant.

VALIDITY OF THE INVENTORIES

Face Validity

A test is said to have face validity if it appears to measure the targeted domain. Face validity is highly desirable for a parent-report measure, as it facilitates a concerted effort by the parent to complete a CDI form fully and accurately. The professional appearance of the CDI forms encourages the parent to take them seriously. Parents will probably be more influenced, however, by the structure and content of the form. Most parents will want to provide a detailed and full account of their children's communicative skills. Parents will notice that the form samples a wide range of communicative skills in considerable depth. That impression should, in turn, increase the probability that parents will regard the form as presenting an opportunity to portray their children's communicative skills accurately and completely.

Content Validity

Another important type of validity is content validity, defined as the extent to which the content of the scale maps onto the content that the investigator hopes to assess. Content validity is determined by examining the features of an instrument to determine whether the components relate to the skills that the instrument is designed to measure. The case for content validity of the CDIs rests on the assertion that the two forms sample the major features of communicative development across the 8- to 30-month age range. The items within each subscale were drawn from the developmental literature and from suggestions made by parents in response to earlier versions of the instrument. For infants, the major domains include Words Understood, Words Produced, and Actions and Gestures. For toddlers, the two main portions of the form center on Words Produced and Sentences and Grammar. Although some dimensions of communication are not included in the CDIs, notably phonology and most aspects of pragmatics (see Dale, 1996), those that are included are covered comprehensively.

Convergent Validity

Additional evidence of validity rests on the fact that the developmental functions obtained with the various subscales correspond closely to the developmental functions that have been reported for the same variables in observational studies. We regard the close parallels between CDI data and developmental patterns reported in the laboratory as extremely important evidence of validity. Although the parallels between CDI growth curves and patterns reported in the literature do not quite fit the traditional meaning of convergent validity (Anastasi, 1988), the term fits better than do others.

The developmental functions are monotonic (i.e., they increase regularly across the relevant age range), the floor for each measure corresponds closely to the age of onset reported in the literature, and rates of development correspond to longitudinal and cross-sectional findings reported in studies using other techniques. With a few exceptions, the range of variation observed around each function also appears to be quite credible, based on what is known from observational studies. Exceptions include the variation in word comprehension observed at 8 months of age (when approximately 10% of the parents report receptive vocabularies that are much larger than estimates in prior studies) and the very early age of onset of certain types of pretend actions reported by some parents. In these cases, we suspect that some parents have applied a different and more liberal definition of the behavior in question than we had in mind. Overall, however, there appears to be an excellent match between our intent and the parents' interpretations.

We were particularly surprised at the impressive validity obtained with the grammatical assessments contained in Part II of CDI: Words and Sentences for two reasons. First, in contrast with the gestural and lexical assessments obtained with other sections of the two inventories, we had little experience in the use of parental report to assess grammar. Second, some investigators have reported that grammatical and phonological skills are particularly difficult for nonexperts to define and for laymen to think about independent of the particular contexts in which those skills are used (e.g., Gleitman & Gleitman, 1970). In designing the grammatical assessment section of the CDI: Words and Sentences form, we tried to circumvent those problems by using a recognition format in which parents were asked to identify grammatical forms that their child was using or to select sentences matching the level of their child's speech.

The developmental functions obtained for the grammar scales correspond closely to reports in the literature. This finding includes the relative time of onset for word combinations as well as the acceleration in grammatical complexity observed between 18 months (when very few children use grammatical inflections) and 30 months (when most children use a variety of grammatical inflections and function words). It also includes the rank orders observed among specific grammatical morphemes (e.g., noun inflections tend to come in before verb inflections, irregular past tense verbs tend to come in before regular past tense verbs) and the age of onset and relative infrequency of overgeneralizations (i.e., incorrect forms like "foots" and "eated"). Because we can assume that very few parents have textbook knowledge of child language, we conclude that the developmental functions obtained with the CDI forms correspond to reports in the literature because parents and psycholinguists are listening to and reporting the same developmental phenomena.

Despite this evidence for convergent validity, it is also important to determine whether the scores obtained for individual children with the CDIs correspond to scores the same children would obtain in laboratory testing and/or home observations. This brings us to correlational studies of the concurrent and predictive validity of the CDIs and their predecessors.

Concurrent Validity

Concurrent validity was determined by assessing the relation between parent report (i.e., CDI scores) and child performance on standardized and laboratory measures of the relevant dimension of language development. One of the major motivations for developing the CDIs was the need for improved measures of language abilities in this difficult-to-test age range. Thus, validity correlations for CDI measures are likely to be limited by the reliability and validity of the criterion measures. In the following summary, we concentrate on the core CDI measures—specifically, Words Understood, Words Produced, and Total Gestures on the CDI: Words and Gestures form and Words Produced, Complexity, and Examples/M3L on the CDI: Words and Sentences form. Some of the studies listed provide validity information on other CDI measures as well. These areas are discussed as part of the following broader areas: vocabulary, gestural communication, grammatical development.

Vocabulary   Because the vocabulary checklists in the inventories are little changed from earlier versions, evidence of concurrent validity of the earlier forms generalizes to the new CDI forms. In particular, we include studies of the validity of the vocabulary checklists included in the Language and Gestures Inventory (precursor of the CDI: Words and Gestures) and the Early Language Inventory (precursor of the CDI: Words and Sentences), although not earlier versions.

A summary of correlational validity studies for vocabulary for these instruments is presented in Table 4.34. The correlations between laboratory measures and inventory scores are generally substantial, and they are highest for the most valid and specific criterion variables: observed vocabulary and the Expressive One Word Picture Vocabulary Test (EOWPVT).

In the two Dale (1990, 1991) studies reported in Table 4.34, scores on the CDI: Words and Sentences vocabulary scale were compared with laboratory assessments carried out on a group of toddlers drawn from the larger norming sample, within 1 month following the parent's completion of the toddler inventory. Although correlations between the laboratory measures and the children's scores on the CDI were substantial (.53 to .73), Dale (1991) argued that limitations of the criterion measures may nonetheless lead to underestimates of the true validity of the CDI vocabulary scale. He noted that the EOWPVT is primarily a measure of concrete noun vocabulary, whereas the Type–Token Ratio (derived from a language sample) is particularly sensitive to high-frequency words. Hence, each of these measures may effectively index only a portion of the child's semantic knowledge. In support of this argument, the multiple correlation (R) between children's scores on the CDI: Words and Sentences Vocabulary scale and the two observational measures together is $R = .79$ $(p < .001)$, which is higher than either simple correlation. Thus, the CDI: Words and Sentences Vocabulary checklist appears to assess a broader vocabulary range than either of the individual direct observation measures.

Table 4.34 reports only the English data from Marchman & Martínez-Sussmann's (2002) study of English-Spanish bilingual children. Their measures also included the Mexican Spanish adaptation of the CDIs (Jackson-Maldonado et al., 2003), as well as language sample measures parallel to those in English. The validity correlations for Spanish were quite similar to those for English. Moreover, their analyses demonstrated that parents are "able to accurately discriminate children's English and Spanish word use when completing the [CDIs], even if they were speakers of both English and Spanish themselves" (p. 994).

Stallings et al. (2002) and Thal et al. (2006—under review) evaluated CDI measures from children with severe to profound deafness who have received cochlear implants. Although children who are eligible for implants are substantially beyond the design age range of the CDIs, their language development to a great extent really begins at implantation. Stallings et al. instructed parents to mark a word as *understands and says* if the child could sign and/or vocalize the word and to mark the word as *understands* if the child understood the word in signed and/or spoken form. In their study, the CDI: Words and Gestures and CDI: Words and Sentences data were obtained from different families. In the Thal et al. study, because the length of implant use varied considerably, it was not clear which form would be more appropriate; therefore, mothers were asked to complete both forms. Another contrast with the Stallings et al. study is that mothers were asked to mark only oral English forms understood or used, not signed forms. Despite these differences, the results of the two studies were quite comparable. (Both studies provide considerable additional information on the validity of the CDI measures beyond the summary provided here.)

In addition to these correlational studies, several other studies have compared vocabulary scores with other measures with alternative statistical analyses. Thal and Bates (1988) showed that parent report of production and comprehension, assessed by the Language and Gesture Inventory, corresponds to laboratory measures of the same language skills. In this study, language comprehension and production of a group of language delayed 18- to 28-month-old toddlers were sampled, using the Language and Gesture Inventory as the parent-report

Table 4.34. Summary of validity studies regarding parent reports of child vocabulary production and comprehension

Parent-report measure	Laboratory measure	Sample Age (in months)	Sample Description	N	r	Study source (see table note)
Production						
Language and Gesture Inventory: Production	Language sample NDW	13	Unselected	27	.72	1
CDI: Words and Gestures	Language sample NDW	24–32	Language delayed	12	.66	6
	Preschool Language Scale–Revised (PLS-R; Zimmerman, Steiner, & Pond, 1979)	24–32	Language delayed	12	.52	6
CDI: Words and Gestures	Peabody Picture Vocabulary Test, Third Edition (PPVT-III; Dunn & Dunn, 1997)	17–72	6 months post-cochlear implantation	28	.67	13
	Reynell Developmental Language Scales (RDLS) Expressive (Reynell & Gruber, 1990)	17–72	6 months post-cochlear implantation	29	.75	13
CDI: Words and Gestures	RDLS Expressive	30–86	3–60 mos. post-cochlear implantation	32	.82	14
	Language sample NDW[a]	30–86	3–60 mos. post-cochlear implantation	32	.77	14
Early Language Inventory	Language sample NDW	20	Unselected	27	.83	1
Early Language Inventory	Bayley Scales of Infant Development–Second Edition: Expressive Language Scale (Bayley, 1993)[b]	20[c]	Full term	32	.59	2
	Bayley Language scale[b]	20[c]	Preterm	21	.33	2
	Bayley Language scale[b]	20[c]	Social risk	65	.48	2
	Bayley Language scale[b]	20[c]	Precocious	44	.63	2
Early Language Inventory	Language sample Word Roots[d]	20	Unselected	187	.60	7
	British Edition of the RDLS (Reynell & Huntley,1985)[e]	20	Unselected	187	.78	7
Early Language Inventory	Bayley Expressive Language[b]	25	Unselected	42	.56	3
	Language sample NDW	25	Unselected	42	.79	3
CDI: Words and Sentences	Preschool Language Scale–Revised (PLS-R; Zimmerman, Steiner, & Pond, 1979)	20	Unselected	20	.40	4
CDI: Words and Sentences	PLS-R Vocabulary subscale	29	Unselected	20	.61	4
	Language sample NDW-50[f]	20	Unselected	20	.67	4
CDI: Words and Sentences	Expressive One-Word Picture Vocabulary Test (EOWPVT; Gardner, 1981)	24	Unselected	24	.73	5
CDI: Words and Sentences	Language sample NDW-100[g]	24	Unselected	24	.53	5
CDI: Words and Sentences	EOWPVT	39–49	Language impaired	20	.86	6
	Language sample NDW-100U[h]	39–49	Language impaired	20	.78	6
CDI: Words and Sentences	Bayley Expressive Language[b]	33[i]	Down syndrome	44	.77	8
	Language sample NDW	33[i]	Down syndrome	44	.82	8
CDI: Words and Sentences	Bayley Expressive Language[b]	17[i]	Typically developing	46	.70	8
	Language sample NDW	17[i]	Typically developing	46	.75	8

CDI: Words and Sentences	Sequenced Inventory of Communication Development–Revised Edition (SICD-R; Hedrick, Prather, & Tobin, 1984)	Autism spectrum disorder	24	31	.55	10
CDI: Words and Sentences	Verbal recall of event[i]	Unselected	24	24–48	.55	11
CDI: Words and Sentences	Language sample NDW[k]	Bilingual English-Spanish	28	26	.79	12
CDI: Words and Sentences	Object naming[l]	Bilingual English-Spanish	28	26	.72	12
CDI: Words and Sentences	PPVT-III	12 months post-cochlear implantation	38–67	17	.64	13
CDI: Words and Sentences	RDLS Expressive	12 months post-cochlear implantation	38–67	18	.87	13
CDI: Words and Sentences	RDLS Expressive	3–60 months post-cochlear implantation	30–86	32	.88	14
CDI: Words and Sentences	Language sample NDW[a]	3–60 months post-cochlear implantation	30–86	32	.74	14
Comprehension						
Language and Gesture Inventory: Comprehension	Multiple-choice object	Unselected		27	.52	1
CDI: Words and Gestures	Picture identification task	Language delayed	24–32	12	.51[m]	6
CDI: Words and Gestures	Index of Productive Syntax (IPSyn; Scarborough, 1990)[j]	Unselected	12	11	.78	9
CDI: Words and Gestures	Index of Productive Syntax[n]	Unselected	18	11	.87	9
CDI: Words and Gestures	PPVT-III	6 months post-cochlear implantation	17–72	28	.56	13
CDI: Words and Gestures	RDLS Receptive	6 months post-cochlear implantation	17–72	29	.59	13
CDI: Words and Gestures	RDLS Receptive	3–60 months post-cochlear implantation	30–86	32	.6	14
CDI: Words and Gestures	Language sample NDW[a]	3–60 months post-cochlear implantation	30–86	32	.72	14

Sources: 1. Bates, Bretherton, & Snyder (1988); 2. Dale, Bates, Reznick, & Morisset (1989); 3. Beeghly, Jernberg, & Burrows (1989); 4. Dale (1991); 5. Dale (1990); 6. Thal, O'Hanlon, Clemmons, & Fralin (1999); 7. Bornstein & Haynes (1998); 8. Miller, Sedey, & Miolo (1995); 9. Rollins (2003); 10. Stone & Yoder (2001); 11. Simcock & Hayne (2003); 12. Marchman & Martinez-Sussmann (2002); 13. Stallings, Gao, & Svirsky (2002); 14. Thal, DesJardin, & Eisenberg (2006–under review).

Key: N = total number in sample; r = Pearson product–moment correlation; NDW = number of different words.

a NDW based on a 7–10 minute language sample, including free play and joint book reading with parent.
b For details on the Bayley Language and Expressive Language subscales, see Dale, P.S., Bates, E., Reznick, S., & Morisset, C. (1989).
c Bayley Scales administered 4 months later, at 24 months.
d Number of different word roots based on 10-minute language sample.
e As opposed to the U.S. Edition.
f NDW based on 50 tokens; subjects with fewer productions omitted.
g NDW based on 100 tokens; subjects with fewer productions omitted.
h NDW based on 100 utterances.
i Verbal recall assessed 24 hours following a structured interaction with the "Magic Shrinking Machine."
j Down syndrome and typically developing group were both selected to be functioning at approximately the 20-month cognitive age level.
k NDW based on 24-minute language sample, part with parent and part with research assistant.
l Naming of 15 common objects.
m Nonsignificant due to small sample size.
n IPSyn based on language sample obtained at 30 months.

measure. Laboratory measures were based on a spontaneous language sample (for production) and a forced-choice picture identification task (for comprehension). The children's vocabulary comprehension scores on the Language and Gesture Inventory were significantly higher than their production scores. The same disparity was seen for the laboratory measures.

In another study, Bates and colleagues (1989) compared parental report of comprehension in 12- to 16-month-old children with measures of the extent to which the children used adult speech cues in an imitation task. Children were asked to imitate a recognitory gesture, such as drinking, while holding a neutral object (a block). The modeled gestures were accompanied by language that was either supportive, neutral, or contradictory. For example, when modeling a drinking gesture, the experimenter might have said, "Look at the cup" (supportive language), "Look at this" (neutral language), or "Look at the baby" (contradictory language). Children were divided into low-, middle-, and high-comprehension groups (based on the Language and Gesture Inventory). Children with low comprehension showed no effect of language support; children with middle-level comprehension were helped by supportive language but showed no effect for neutral or contradictory language; and children with high comprehension performed well with supportive and neutral language but did poorly with contradictory language. Thus, parental report of vocabulary comprehension predicted how children used language input in an experimental task.

Nott, Cowan, Brown, and Wigglesworth (2003) assessed the language development of nine children with congenital severe to profound sensorineural hearing loss who attended an oral/auditory early intervention program. Initial assessment occurred during the second year of life, and follow-up assessments occurred approximately every 6 months thereafter. The instruments included the Vocabulary Production component of the CDI: Words and Gestures or the CDI: Words and Sentences, the Rossetti Infant-Toddler Language Scale, and a specially developed parental diary system (Di-EL) designed to capture all of the child's first 100 utterances. The scores of the three tools were highly correlated after 12 months of device (hearing aid or cochlear implant) use: $r = .99$ for the CDI and the Rossetti Infant-Toddler Language Scale and $r = .98$ for the CDI and the Di-EL. (The exact ages involved are not reported.) The authors also compared the two parent-report measures at the level of individual words. The percentage of agreement (occurrence/nonoccurrence) ranged from 87 to 96 for the nine children, and the corresponding Kappa values (k) ranged from .63 to .81. As might be expected, a common phenomenon was the occurrence of words in the parental diary that were not on the CDI list.

Gestural Communication Because of a lack of standardized, accepted measures of gestural communication that can serve as a criterion measure, few correlational studies similar to those discussed in the previous section are available for this measure. Carpenter, Nagell, and Tomasello (1998) evaluated social and communicative development between 9 and 15 months in a sample of 24 children. They compared scores on Part II, Section A (First Communicative Gestures) of the CDI: Words and Gestures with a laboratory-based measure of joint attention between mother and infant during a 10-minute free-play period. It is interesting to note that the relation peaked at approximately 11–13 months: of the nine correlations between joint attention at 11, 12, and 13 months and gestural communication at the same ages, five were significant, ranging from .43 to .62. Thal and colleagues (1999) compared CDI: Words and Gestures total number of gestures produced (summing Part II Sections A through E) with a gesture imitation task that had been developed by Bates et al. (1989) to measure production of recognitory gestures. The correlation in their sample of 12 24- to 32-month-old children with language delay was a weak and nonsignificant .30. As Thal et al. pointed out, the range of gestures on the CDI: Words and Gestures is much wider than in their direct test, and this may have reduced the correlation. Yet, the total number of gestures that parents reported on the CDI: Words and Gestures did correlate strongly (.65) with Preschool Language Scale–Revised (PLS-R; Zimmerman, Steiner, & Pond, 1979) language comprehension age, consistent with much other evidence for a close relation between gestures and language comprehension in this age range.

Several other studies have been conducted to validate Part II of the CDI: Words and Gestures form, including preverbal communicative gestures and routines (sections A and B) and recognitory or symbolic gestures with objects (Sections C through E), using alternative designs. These studies also provided some additional validation of the word comprehension measures on the CDI: Words and Gestures (Part I).

Thal and Hoffman (1990) selected groups of children from the norming study who fell at the high or low end of the distribution on total number of gestures reported (summing across Part II, Sections A through E). Eighteen children with high gesture scores and 16 children with low gesture scores participated in a laboratory study conducted 3–5 months after their parents had completed a CDI: Words and Gestures form. For statistical analysis, children were divided into three age groups on the basis of age at laboratory assessment: 11–13 months, 14–16 months, and 17–21 months. Laboratory measures included assessments of spontaneous symbolic play (i.e., recognitory gestures with familiar objects), elicitation of recognitory gestures under a range of conditions (after Thal & Bates, 1988), two forced-choice word comprehension tasks (one with pairs of pictures, another with sets of real objects), and a task designed to elicit gestural requests and indications of objects (after Snyder, 1975). There were significant differences between the high- and low-gesture groups at the first two age levels on all laboratory symbolic/recognitory gesture measures. There were also significant differences as reported on the CDI: Words and Gestures form and observed on the word comprehension task, supporting the high correlations between gestures and word comprehension reported in other studies (e.g., Bates et al., 1989) and for the norming sample as a whole. This finding can also be regarded as a partial validation of the CDI: Words and Gestures Words Understood scale. No differences were found on the Snyder Gestural Communication task.

Thal and Dughi (1990) conducted a longitudinal study of 12 infants between 8 and 12 months of age (an unselected and normally distributed sample in contrast with the stratified sample studied by Thal & Hoffman, 1990). Parents completed the CDI: Words and Gestures form at monthly intervals across the 8- to 12-month range. At 10 and again at 12 months of age, children participated in laboratory sessions using the previously described assessments of communicative gestures, recognitory or symbolic gestures, and word comprehension. Correlations between laboratory and parental report scales were calculated within the respective 10- and 12-month levels to establish concurrent validity; short-term predictive validity was assessed through correlations between the 10-month CDI subscales and the 12-month laboratory measures. In addition, 10- to 12-month correlations were obtained for the CDI to examine its stability across a 2-month period. There were substantial and significant concurrent correlations between the infant form Gesture scores and laboratory measures of spontaneous and elicited symbolic play at 12 months of age. At 10 months, concurrent validity was found only for First Communicative Gestures (Part II, Section A). However, parental report of symbolic/recognitory gestures at 10 months did show significant predictive correlations with laboratory observations of the same activities 2 months later. In addition, parental reports of recognitory gestures at both ages predicted observations of spontaneous naming at the 12-month level. These gesture-to-language correlations were particularly large, ranging from .71 (from 10-month gestures to 12-month naming) to .82 (for 12-month gestures with 12-month naming). Within-language correlations included a .90 relation between reported and observed naming at 12 months.

Grammatical Development   Table 4.35 summarizes the results of correlational validity studies of Part II, Sections D and E of the CDI: Words and Sentences form. The data for the first three entries are drawn from the studies described in the previous section reporting the validity of the vocabulary measures of the two inventories. In each study, a 100-word utterance language sample was videotaped during a free-play session with the child and his or her mother. The sample was transcribed and scored for MLU using an expansion of the procedures recommended by Miller (1981). The correlations between the Complexity scale and MLU were very high ($r = .88$ and $.76$ for 20- and 24-month-olds, respectively). The correlations between M3L provided by the parent and the laboratory MLU were also very high ($r = .77$ and $.74$ for the 20- and 24-month-olds, respectively). Thus, both of the CDI: Words and Sentences measures of grammatical development (Complexity and Examples/M3L) were excellent predictors of observed MLU. These validity correlations are nearly as high as the reliability of MLU itself, estimated by Dale (1990) to be approximately .80. Therefore, nearly all of the reliable variance in MLU is captured by the CDI: Words and Sentences. The validity of these measures for a group of young children with language impairment (Thal et al., 1999) is lower but still substantial. The figures are slightly lower still for the bilingual sample studied by Marchman and Martínez-Sussmann (2002). A comparison of those cases in which the same reporters filled out the CDIs for both languages versus that in which different reporters filled out one in each language suggested that bilingual reporters may have some difficulty discriminating grammatical development in the two languages, unlike the situation for vocabulary discussed previously in this section.

Table 4.35.   Summary of validity studies regarding parent reports of child sentence complexity and three longest sentences

Parent-report measure (all sections from Part 2 of CDI: Words and Sentences)	Laboratory measure	Sample					
		Age (in months)	Description	N	r	Source	
Sentence Complexity (Section E)	MLU 100-utterance sample	20	Unselected	20	.88	1	
Max Sentence Length (Section D)	MLU 100-utterance sample	20	Unselected	20	.77	1	
Sentence Complexity (Section E)	MLU 100-utterance sample	24	Unselected	24	.76	2	
Max Sentence Length (Section D)	MLU 100-utterance sample	24	Unselected	24	.74	2	
Sentence Complexity (Section E)	MLU 100-utterance sample	39–49	Language impaired	20	.69	3	
Max Sentence Length (Section D)	MLU 100-utterance sample	39–49	Language impaired	20	.63	3	
Sentence Complexity (Section E)	MLU[a]	28	Bilingual English-Spanish	26	.64	4	
Max Sentence Length (Section D)	MLU[a]	28	Bilingual English-Spanish	26	.53	4	
Sentence Complexity (Section E)	Reynell Developmental Language Scales (RDLS)–Third Edition: Expressive (Edwards et al., 1997)	38–67	12 months post-cochlear implantation	18	.89	5	
Max Sentence Length (Section D)	RDLS Expressive	38–67	12 months post-cochlear implantation	18	.73	5	
Sentence Complexity (Section E)	MLU[b]	30–86	3–60 months post-cochlear implantation	32	.61	6	
Max Sentence Length (Section D)	MLU[b]	30–86	3–60 months post-cochlear implantation	32	.64	6	

Sources: 1. Dale (1990); 2. Dale (1991); 3. O'Hanlon & Thal (1991); 4. Marchman & Martínez-Sussmann (2002); 5. Stallings, Gao, & Svirsky (2002); 6. Thal, DesJardin, & Eisenberg (2006–under review).

Key: N = total number in sample; *r* = Pearson product–moment correlation; MLU = mean length of utterance.

[a]MLU in words, based on 24-minute language sample, part with parent and part with research assistant

[b]MLU based on a 7–10 minute language sample including free play and joint book reading with parent

Predictive Validity

An instrument possesses predictive validity to the extent that components of the instrument measured at one point in time correlate with the same or other components of the instrument or to other measures of the same construct measured at subsequent points in time. (Sometimes the term *predictive validity* is used for any predictive correlation with a later, theoretically salient measure, such as the prediction from early language to reading. We consider such studies to be more appropriately viewed as substantive research on developmental processes rather than validity per se.) Research with the predecessors of the CDIs provided substantial evidence for the predictive power of parent-report instruments across the first 3 years of life (Bates et al., 1979; Bates et al., 1988; Dale et al., 1989). For example, Bates et al., (1988) found correlations in the range of .60 to .80 between estimates of productive vocabulary at 20 months (using parent report) and various measures of vocabulary and grammar at 28 months (using observational data).

The CDI norming study involved the reassessment of a relatively large number of children. Their parents completed a second CDI approximately 6 months after filling out the first questionnaire. Because two forms, the CDI: Words and Gestures and the CDI: Words and Sentences, are used to span the age range from 8 to 30 months, the parents may have completed the same CDI both times or may have completed one CDI at Time 1 and another at Time 2. As a result, the longitudinal data include three subgroups, to be discussed in turn:

1.   CDI: Words and Sentences to CDI: Words and Sentences

2.   CDI: Words and Gestures to CDI: Words and Sentences

3.   CDI: Words and Gestures to CDI: Words and Gestures

These data provide further evidence on the predictive validity of the CDIs. Because some of the measures administered at Times 1 and 2 were either identical or similar, these data may also be regarded as a measure of reliability.

Parents of 228 children completed the CDI: Words and Sentences for a second time. At Time 1, the children ranged in age from 16 to 24 months; at Time 2, from 22 to 30 months. The total vocabulary scores at Times 1 and 2 were correlated at .71 ($p < .0001$). To remove age-based variance, a series of separate correlations were computed within each Time 1 age level. All correlations remained significant and relatively large. It is interesting to note that an inverted U-shaped pattern was obtained between the size of the correlation and age in the early portion of the age range. The values for successive Time 1 ages from 16 to 21 months were .53, .58, .66, .73, .81, and .70. From 22 to 24 months, the correlation was .74 or greater at each monthly age level. In line with earlier findings by Bates et al. (1988), 20 months of age appears to be the point at which estimates of total vocabulary by parental report yield their maximum predictive power. Nevertheless, the correlations are substantial and reasonably stable across the entire age range spanned by the CDI: Words and Sentences.

The same data set was used to examine the 6-month stability of Complexity scores. The simple correlation between Time 1 and Time 2 scores was .62 ($p = .0001$). Again, to control for age, a series of separate correlations was computed within each Time 1 age level. These correlations were lower for children with Time 1 ages of younger than 20 months, due to the reduced variation in grammatical complexity scores. Indeed, the Time 1-Time 2 correlation at 16 months was a nonsignificant .16. The correlations from 17 to 19 months were .50, .47, and .50, respectively ($p < .01$ in each case). From 20 months to 24 months (the oldest group included at Time 1), higher correlations were obtained: .65, .62, .62, .62, and .60, respectively.

Parents of another 217 children completed the CDI: Words and Gestures at Time 1, when their children were between 10 and 16 months of age, and the CDI: Words and Sentences at Time 2, when their ages ranged from 16 to 25 months. The correlation between Time 1 and Time 2 total vocabulary production scores (the one measure derivable from both forms) was .69 ($p < .0001$). To control for age, separate correlations were computed for five age groups: 10–11, 12, 13, 14, and 15–16 months. Combining ages in this way yielded sample sizes of 34–51 children per group. The resulting correlations (all significant) were .65, .38, .69, .70, and 73, respectively. With the exception of the 12-month group, these scores indicate impressive cross-form, cross-age stability from the early period of vocabulary development to a period of more rapid vocabulary expansion. It is interesting to note that the high variability reflected by the lower 12-month value is consistent with the results of our 6-week reliability test–retest assessment of the CDI: Words and Gestures, which was conducted with a different subsample. As reported in the section on reliability, a dramatic drop in stability occurred between 12 and 13 months, relative to the months preceding and following that point in age, and is perhaps attributable to a developmental transition that occurs at approximately 12 months.

Finally, parents of 62 children completed the CDI: Words and Gestures twice, first when their children were between 8 and 10 months of age, and again when their children were between 14 and 17 months old. Because the age span for these data was restricted, we did not calculate separate correlations by month with raw scores or z scores. Rather, we obtained overall longitudinal correlations for the major components of the inventory. For total vocabulary production, the correlation was .38 ($p < .01$). The longitudinal correlations were slightly higher for total vocabulary comprehension (.44, $p < .001$) and for total gestures (.44, $p < .01$). These results provide some evidence for predictive validity within the 8- to 16-month range for the major components of the CDI: Words and Gestures. However, it is also clear that these scores show less overall stability at younger than 11 months of age, compared with the CDI: Words and Sentences to CDI: Words and Sentences and the CDI: Words and Gestures to CDI: Words and Sentences correspondences previously reported in this chapter.

The conclusions of the predictive component of the CDI norming study, particularly a substantial rise in predictive validity during the second year of life, is supported by several more recent longitudinal studies. Feldman et al. (2000) administered the CDI: Words and Gestures and CDI: Words and Sentences at 1 and 2 years of age, respectively, to a large ($N = 2,156$) and sociodemographically diverse sample. Although the correlations from CDI: Words and Gestures Phrases Understood, Words Understood, and Words Produced to CDI: Words and Sentences Vocabulary Production, Examples/M3L, and Complexity were all significant, they were modest in size. The largest correlation was .39 between Word Produced at the two ages. Feldman et al. suggested that this modest stability is a psychometric defect in the measure. However, Fenson, Bates, and colleagues (2000) pointed out that this result is likely to be an authentic reflection of developmental processes and that even laboratory measures of language development across the second year of life have little stability. In a longitudinal study of 26 children, Bauer, Goldfield, and Reznick (2002) compared the effectiveness of CDI: Words and Gestures Words Produced and Words Understood scores at 8 through 14 months as predictors of CDI: Words and Sentences Words Produced at 21 months. Vocabulary Comprehension scores yielded relatively constant predictive correlations in the range of .25 to .40 across this age range. In contrast, the prediction from Words Produced scores steadily increased from $-.27$ at 8 months to $.84$ at 14 months, becoming statistically significant first at 11 months ($r = .45$) and remaining so thereafter.

Stronger predictions were found across the third year of life by Feldman et al. (2005), who administered the CDI: Words and Sentences and the CDI-III (discussed in Chapter 6) to 113 children at ages 2 and 3 years, respectively. CDI: Words and Sentences Words Produced and CDI-III Vocabulary scores were correlated at $.58$ ($p < .01$). CDI-III Complexity was predicted at $r = .54$ and $.37$ (both $p < .01$) by CDI: Words and Sentences Examples/M3L and Complexity, respectively.

LOOKING AHEAD

There is now a large body of evidence supporting the reliability, validity, clinical utility, and research potential of the MacArthur-Bates Communicative Development Inventories. This success has led our research team and others to further expand these parent report tools. Short forms of both the CDI: Words and Gestures form and the CDI: Words and Sentences form have been developed for applications in research and educational settings where use of the complete forms is not feasible. An upward extension of the CDI: Words and Sentences form for 30- to 37-month-olds, the CDI-III, has also been developed (see Chapter 6). We are designing a specialized form that will be maximally sensitive at the low end of the spectrum, to be used for as a screening measure identifying children at risk for language delay. We hope to establishing a data archive for CDI results from many different research and clinical settings, an initiative that will permit the compilation of "sub-norms" from a range of normal and abnormal populations (e.g., for twins, children from low socioeconomic groups, preterm babies, children with Down syndrome, babies exposed to cocaine and other neurotoxic drugs, young children with cleft palates). Although there are some clear limitations to the use of parent report data, the CDI instruments are finding many useful applications in laboratories, schools, and clinics throughout the United States and other English-speaking countries (with minor modifications as needed for other English dialects such as British, Australian, and New Zealand). In addition, as described previously, many foreign language versions are under development or in use in a variety of settings in the United States and other countries.

5

PERCENTILE TABLES AND FIGURES

These percentile tables and figures are fitted values derived from data collected for the norming of the CDIs. See Chapter 2 for detailed instructions on scoring the CDIs and creating Child Report Forms.

Table 5.1. Fitted percentile scores for Phrases Understood (CDI: Words and Gestures)—both sexes combined

%ile rank	Age (in months)										
	8	9	10	11	12	13	14	15	16	17	18
99	27	27	27	27	28	28	28	28	28	28	28
95	21	23	24	25	26	27	27	28	28	28	28
90	16	19	21	23	24	26	27	27	28	28	28
85	14	16	19	21	23	24	26	27	27	28	28
80	12	15	17	20	22	24	25	26	27	27	28
75	11	13	16	18	21	22	24	25	26	27	28
70	9	11	14	17	19	21	23	25	26	27	27
65	9	11	13	16	18	20	22	24	25	26	27
60	8	10	12	14	17	19	21	22	24	25	26
55	7	9	11	13	16	18	20	22	24	25	26
50	7	9	10	13	15	17	19	21	22	24	25
45	6	7	9	11	14	16	18	20	22	24	25
40	5	7	9	11	13	15	17	19	21	22	24
35	5	6	8	10	12	14	16	18	20	22	23
30	4	6	7	9	11	13	15	17	19	21	23
25	4	5	6	8	9	11	14	16	18	20	22
20	3	4	5	6	8	10	12	14	16	18	20
15	2	3	3	4	6	7	9	12	14	16	18
10	2	2	3	4	5	6	7	9	11	13	16
5	0	0	1	1	2	3	4	6	9	12	15

Table 5.2. Fitted percentile scores for Phrases Understood (CDI: Words and Gestures)—girls

%ile rank	Age (in months)										
	8	9	10	11	12	13	14	15	16	17	18
99	27	27	27	27	27	28	28	28	28	28	28
95	23	24	25	26	26	27	27	28	28	28	28
90	18	20	22	24	25	26	27	27	28	28	28
85	15	18	20	22	24	25	26	27	28	28	28
80	13	16	19	21	23	25	26	27	27	28	28
75	12	15	17	20	22	23	25	26	27	27	28
70	10	12	15	18	20	23	24	26	27	27	28
65	9	11	14	16	19	21	23	25	26	27	27
60	8	11	13	15	18	20	22	24	25	26	27
55	8	10	12	14	17	19	21	23	24	25	26
50	7	9	11	13	15	18	20	22	23	25	26
45	6	8	10	12	14	17	19	21	23	24	25
40	5	7	9	11	13	16	18	20	22	24	25
35	5	6	8	10	12	15	17	19	21	23	24
30	5	6	8	10	12	14	16	18	20	22	24
25	4	5	6	8	10	12	15	17	19	21	23
20	3	4	6	7	9	11	13	15	17	19	21
15	2	3	4	5	7	8	10	13	15	17	19
10	1	2	2	3	4	6	7	9	11	14	16
5	0	0	1	1	1	2	3	5	7	10	13

Table 5.3. Fitted percentile scores for Phrases Understood (CDI: Words and Gestures)—boys

%ile rank	Age (in months)										
	8	9	10	11	12	13	14	15	16	17	18
99	25	26	26	27	27	27	28	28	28	28	28
95	20	22	24	25	26	26	27	27	28	28	28
90	15	17	20	22	23	25	26	27	27	28	28
85	13	16	18	20	22	24	25	26	27	27	28
80	11	14	16	19	21	23	24	25	26	27	28
75	10	13	15	17	19	21	23	25	26	26	27
70	9	11	13	16	18	20	22	24	25	26	27
65	9	11	13	15	17	19	21	23	24	25	26
60	8	9	12	14	16	18	20	22	24	25	26
55	7	9	11	13	15	17	19	21	23	24	25
50	6	8	10	12	14	16	18	20	22	23	25
45	5	7	9	11	13	15	17	19	21	23	24
40	5	7	8	10	12	14	16	18	20	22	23
35	4	6	7	9	11	13	15	17	19	21	23
30	4	5	6	8	10	12	14	16	18	20	22
25	3	4	5	6	8	10	12	14	16	18	20
20	3	3	4	5	7	8	10	12	14	16	18
15	2	2	3	4	5	7	9	11	13	16	18
10	2	2	3	4	4	6	7	9	10	12	14
5	0	0	0	1	1	2	3	4	6	9	12

Table 5.4. Fitted percentile scores for Words Understood (CDI: Words and Gestures)—both sexes combined

%ile rank	Age (in months)										
	8	9	10	11	12	13	14	15	16	17	18
99	276	310	338	357	371	380	386	390	393	394	395
95	122	151	182	213	244	273	299	320	338	353	364
90	81	106	134	166	199	233	264	292	316	336	352
85	65	85	109	137	168	201	233	264	292	315	335
80	52	70	91	117	146	178	212	244	275	301	323
75	45	60	79	103	131	162	196	229	261	289	314
70	37	50	68	90	116	147	180	214	248	279	305
65	32	44	60	79	103	132	164	197	231	263	292
60	28	39	53	70	93	119	150	183	217	250	280
55	24	33	45	61	81	106	136	169	203	238	270
50	21	29	40	55	74	97	126	158	192	227	260
45	18	25	35	48	66	88	116	148	183	219	254
40	16	22	31	43	59	80	106	137	171	207	243
35	13	19	27	38	53	72	96	125	159	195	231
30	12	17	24	33	46	63	85	111	142	177	213
25	11	15	21	29	40	55	74	98	127	159	194
20	10	13	19	26	35	48	65	85	111	140	172
15	7	10	15	21	29	40	54	73	97	125	157
10	5	7	10	15	21	30	41	57	77	103	133
5	2	4	5	8	12	18	26	38	54	76	104

Table 5.5. Fitted percentile scores for Words Understood (CDI: Words and Gestures)—girls

%ile rank	Age (in months)										
	8	9	10	11	12	13	14	15	16	17	18
99	292	324	348	364	376	383	388	391	393	395	396
95	153	195	237	276	309	335	354	368	378	384	389
90	91	117	148	182	216	250	280	307	329	346	360
85	75	97	125	155	188	222	254	283	309	330	347
80	59	79	103	132	163	197	231	263	292	316	336
75	44	60	81	108	139	174	210	246	278	306	330
70	39	54	73	97	126	159	194	229	263	293	318
65	34	48	65	87	114	146	180	216	251	283	310
60	29	40	56	76	101	131	164	201	237	270	300
55	25	36	49	67	90	118	151	186	222	257	288
50	22	31	43	60	82	109	141	176	213	250	282
45	19	27	38	53	72	96	125	158	194	230	264
40	16	23	33	46	63	86	114	148	184	221	257
35	15	21	30	42	58	78	105	136	170	207	243
30	13	19	26	37	51	69	93	121	154	189	225
25	12	17	24	33	46	63	84	110	141	176	211
20	11	15	20	28	39	53	71	93	120	150	184
15	10	13	18	24	33	44	58	76	98	124	153
10	6	8	12	17	23	32	44	60	80	104	133
5	3	4	6	9	14	21	31	45	66	93	126

Table 5.6. Fitted percentile scores for Words Understood (CDI: Words and Gestures)—boys

%ile rank	Age (in months)										
	8	9	10	11	12	13	14	15	16	17	18
99	168	197	226	254	280	303	322	338	352	362	371
95	119	146	174	204	233	261	286	308	327	343	355
90	76	97	121	148	178	208	238	266	292	314	332
85	58	76	98	123	152	183	214	245	274	299	321
80	48	64	83	107	134	164	196	228	258	286	310
75	41	55	73	94	119	148	179	211	243	272	298
70	36	48	64	83	106	132	162	194	225	256	283
65	30	41	55	72	93	118	147	178	211	242	272
60	26	36	48	63	83	106	133	164	196	228	259
55	22	31	42	56	75	97	124	155	188	221	254
50	19	26	36	49	66	87	113	143	176	211	244
45	16	22	31	43	59	79	105	135	168	204	239
40	14	20	28	39	54	73	97	126	158	193	228
35	13	18	26	36	49	66	88	115	146	179	214
30	12	16	23	32	44	60	80	105	135	169	204
25	9	13	18	26	36	50	68	90	118	150	185
20	8	11	16	22	31	43	59	79	104	134	167
15	6	9	12	18	26	36	50	69	94	123	157
10	4	6	9	13	18	25	36	49	67	90	117
5	2	3	5	7	10	15	22	32	47	66	92

Table 5.7. Fitted percentile scores for Words Produced (CDI: Words and Gestures)—both sexes combined

%ile rank	Age (in months)										
	8	9	10	11	12	13	14	15	16	17	18
99	16	26	44	72	111	160	216	268	312	344	365
95	7	11	18	28	43	65	96	135	180	227	271
90	5	8	12	19	29	44	66	95	132	176	221
85	4	6	9	14	21	32	47	70	99	136	179
80	3	5	7	11	18	27	40	59	84	117	156
75	2	4	6	9	14	21	32	48	71	100	137
70	2	3	5	7	11	18	27	41	60	86	120
65	2	3	4	6	10	15	23	35	52	75	107
60	1	2	3	4	7	12	19	30	47	72	105
55	1	2	2	4	6	10	15	24	37	67	96
50	0	0	1	2	3	6	11	20	37	64	94
45	0	0	1	1	3	5	10	19	35	62	80
40	0	0	0	1	1	3	7	14	31	60	71
35	0	0	0	0	1	2	5	12	26	54	70
30	0	0	0	0	1	2	4	10	20	42	66
25	0	0	0	0	0	1	3	7	16	35	59
20	0	0	0	0	0	1	2	6	13	30	56
15	0	0	0	0	0	1	1	3	8	20	42
10	0	0	0	0	0	0	1	2	4	10	18
5	0	0	0	0	0	0	0	0	0	1	1

Table 5.8. Fitted percentile scores for Words Produced (CDI: Words and Gestures)—girls

%ile rank	Age (in months)										
	8	9	10	11	12	13	14	15	16	17	18
99	15	26	43	70	107	155	209	262	306	339	362
95	7	11	19	31	51	80	121	170	224	274	314
90	6	10	15	23	36	54	79	112	152	196	241
85	4	7	11	17	26	39	59	85	119	160	204
80	3	5	9	13	21	32	49	72	103	142	186
75	3	4	7	11	17	27	40	60	88	123	165
70	2	4	6	9	14	22	34	52	77	110	151
65	2	3	5	8	12	19	29	45	67	97	134
60	1	2	4	6	9	15	24	38	59	88	126
55	1	2	3	5	8	12	20	32	49	75	110
50	1	2	3	4	7	10	17	26	41	62	91
45	1	2	2	4	6	10	15	23	39	60	79
40	0	0	0	1	2	4	8	18	36	59	78
35	0	0	0	1	1	3	7	16	33	54	74
30	0	0	0	0	1	2	6	13	28	50	69
25	0	0	0	0	1	1	3	9	21	41	63
20	0	0	0	0	0	1	3	7	16	37	55
15	0	0	0	0	0	1	2	6	13	30	48
10	0	0	0	0	0	0	1	2	5	12	28
5	0	0	0	0	0	0	0	0	0	1	2

Table 5.9. Fitted percentile scores for Words Produced (CDI: Words and Gestures)—boys

%ile rank	\multicolumn{11}{c}{Age (in months)}										
	8	9	10	11	12	13	14	15	16	17	18
99	10	16	24	37	55	81	114	155	200	244	284
95	7	11	16	24	36	53	76	105	141	182	225
90	4	7	10	15	23	34	50	72	101	137	177
85	3	5	7	11	17	25	37	53	76	105	141
80	3	4	6	9	14	21	31	45	65	91	124
75	2	3	4	7	10	16	25	39	59	86	122
70	2	3	4	6	9	14	22	33	49	72	102
65	1	2	3	5	8	12	18	27	40	60	89
60	1	2	2	4	6	9	14	22	34	58	85
55	0	0	1	1	3	5	10	19	33	53	83
50	0	0	1	1	2	5	9	17	31	52	81
45	0	0	1	1	2	4	8	14	26	47	74
40	0	0	0	1	1	2	5	12	25	45	71
35	0	0	0	0	1	2	4	10	20	42	66
30	0	0	0	0	1	2	4	8	16	34	56
25	0	0	0	0	0	1	2	5	12	27	50
20	0	0	0	0	0	1	1	4	9	22	41
15	0	0	0	0	0	0	1	2	6	14	32
10	0	0	0	0	0	0	0	1	2	5	12
5	0	0	0	0	0	0	0	0	1	1	3

Table 5.10. Fitted percentile scores for Total Gestures (CDI: Words and Gestures)—both sexes combined

%ile rank	\multicolumn{11}{c}{Age (in months)}										
	8	9	10	11	12	13	14	15	16	17	18
99	36	41	46	50	54	56	58	60	61	62	63
95	24	29	34	39	43	47	51	54	56	58	60
90	20	25	30	35	39	44	48	51	54	56	58
85	19	23	27	32	36	40	44	48	51	54	56
80	17	21	25	30	34	39	43	47	50	53	55
75	15	19	23	27	32	36	41	45	48	51	54
70	14	18	21	26	30	35	39	43	47	50	53
65	13	16	20	24	29	33	38	42	46	49	52
60	12	15	19	23	27	32	36	41	45	48	51
55	12	15	18	22	26	30	35	39	43	47	50
50	11	14	17	21	25	29	34	38	42	46	50
45	10	13	16	19	23	27	32	36	41	45	48
40	9	12	15	18	22	26	31	35	40	44	47
35	9	11	14	17	21	25	29	33	38	42	46
30	8	10	13	16	19	23	28	32	36	41	45
25	7	9	12	15	18	22	27	31	36	40	44
20	6	8	11	13	17	21	25	30	34	39	43
15	6	7	9	12	15	18	22	27	31	36	40
10	5	6	8	10	13	16	20	24	29	33	38
5	4	5	6	8	11	13	17	21	25	29	34

Table 5.11. Fitted percentile scores for Total Gestures (CDI: Words and Gestures)—girls

%ile rank	Age (in months)										
	8	**9**	**10**	**11**	**12**	**13**	**14**	**15**	**16**	**17**	**18**
99	33	39	44	49	52	55	58	60	61	62	62
95	24	29	35	40	45	49	53	56	58	60	61
90	20	25	30	35	41	45	49	53	56	58	59
85	18	23	28	33	38	43	47	51	54	56	58
80	17	22	26	31	36	41	45	49	52	55	57
75	16	20	25	29	34	39	43	47	50	53	56
70	15	19	23	27	32	37	41	45	49	52	55
65	14	18	22	26	30	35	40	44	48	51	54
60	13	16	20	24	29	34	38	43	47	50	53
55	12	15	19	23	28	32	37	41	45	49	52
50	11	14	18	22	26	31	36	40	44	48	52
45	10	13	16	20	25	30	35	39	44	48	51
40	9	12	15	19	24	28	33	38	42	46	50
35	9	11	14	18	22	27	32	37	41	45	49
30	8	10	13	17	21	25	30	35	39	44	47
25	7	9	12	15	19	23	28	33	38	42	46
20	7	9	11	14	18	22	26	31	35	40	44
15	6	7	9	12	15	19	23	28	33	37	42
10	5	6	8	11	14	17	21	25	30	34	39
5	3	4	5	7	9	13	16	21	26	31	37

Table 5.12. Fitted percentile scores for Total Gestures (CDI: Words and Gestures)—boys

%ile rank	Age (in months)										
	8	**9**	**10**	**11**	**12**	**13**	**14**	**15**	**16**	**17**	**18**
99	34	38	42	46	49	52	54	56	58	59	60
95	26	30	34	38	42	45	49	51	54	56	57
90	23	27	31	34	38	42	45	48	51	53	55
85	19	22	26	30	35	39	42	46	49	52	54
80	16	20	24	28	32	36	40	44	48	51	53
75	15	18	22	26	30	34	38	42	46	49	52
70	14	17	21	25	28	32	37	40	44	47	50
65	13	16	19	23	27	31	35	39	43	47	50
60	12	15	18	22	26	30	34	38	42	46	49
55	11	14	17	21	25	29	33	37	41	45	48
50	10	13	16	19	23	27	32	36	40	44	47
45	10	12	15	18	22	26	30	34	38	42	46
40	9	11	14	17	21	25	29	33	37	41	45
35	9	11	13	16	20	24	28	32	36	40	44
30	8	10	12	15	19	23	27	31	36	40	44
25	7	9	11	14	17	21	25	30	34	38	42
20	6	8	10	13	16	20	24	28	33	37	41
15	6	7	9	12	15	18	22	26	30	35	39
10	5	7	8	11	13	16	19	23	27	31	36
5	3	4	5	7	9	12	15	18	22	27	32

Table 5.13.　Fitted percentile scores for Early Gestures (CDI: Words and Gestures)—both sexes combined

%ile rank	Age (in months)										
	8	**9**	**10**	**11**	**12**	**13**	**14**	**15**	**16**	**17**	**18**
99	16	16	17	17	17	18	18	18	18	18	18
95	13	14	15	15	16	16	17	17	18	18	18
90	12	13	14	14	15	16	16	17	17	17	18
85	11	12	12	13	14	15	15	16	16	17	17
80	10	11	12	13	14	15	15	16	16	17	17
75	9	10	11	12	13	14	15	16	16	17	17
70	9	10	11	12	13	14	14	15	16	16	17
65	8	9	10	11	12	13	14	15	15	16	17
60	7	9	10	11	12	13	14	14	15	16	16
55	7	8	9	10	11	12	13	14	15	15	16
50	7	8	9	10	11	12	13	14	15	15	16
45	7	7	8	9	10	11	12	13	14	15	15
40	6	7	8	9	10	11	12	13	14	15	15
35	6	7	8	9	10	11	12	13	13	14	15
30	6	7	7	8	9	10	11	12	13	14	15
25	5	6	7	8	9	10	11	12	13	14	14
20	5	6	6	7	8	9	10	11	12	13	14
15	4	5	6	7	8	9	10	11	12	13	13
10	3	3	4	5	6	7	8	10	11	12	13
5	2	3	4	4	5	6	7	8	10	11	12

Table 5.14.　Fitted percentile scores for Early Gestures (CDI: Words and Gestures)—girls

%ile rank	Age (in months)										
	8	**9**	**10**	**11**	**12**	**13**	**14**	**15**	**16**	**17**	**18**
99	16	16	17	17	17	18	18	18	18	18	18
95	14	15	15	16	17	17	17	18	18	18	18
90	11	13	14	15	15	16	17	17	18	18	18
85	11	12	13	14	15	15	16	17	17	17	18
80	11	12	12	13	14	15	15	16	16	17	17
75	10	11	12	13	14	15	15	16	16	17	17
70	9	10	11	12	13	14	15	16	16	17	17
65	9	10	11	12	13	14	15	15	16	17	17
60	8	9	10	11	12	13	14	15	16	16	17
55	8	9	10	11	12	13	14	15	15	16	16
50	7	8	9	11	12	13	13	14	15	16	16
45	6	8	9	10	11	12	13	14	15	16	16
40	6	7	8	9	11	12	13	14	15	16	16
35	6	7	8	9	10	11	12	13	14	15	16
30	6	7	8	9	10	11	12	13	14	14	15
25	5	6	7	8	9	10	11	13	13	14	15
20	5	6	7	8	9	10	11	12	13	14	14
15	4	5	6	7	8	9	10	11	12	13	14
10	3	4	5	6	7	8	9	10	11	12	13
5	2	2	3	4	5	6	7	9	10	11	13

Table 5.15. Fitted percentile scores for Early Gestures (CDI: Words and Gestures)—boys

%ile rank	Age (in months)										
	8	9	10	11	12	13	14	15	16	17	18
99	15	15	15	16	16	16	17	17	18	18	18
95	13	14	14	15	15	16	16	17	17	18	18
90	11	12	12	13	14	14	15	16	17	18	18
85	10	11	12	12	13	14	15	15	16	17	18
80	9	10	11	11	12	13	14	15	16	17	18
75	9	9	10	11	12	13	14	15	16	17	18
70	8	9	10	10	11	12	13	14	15	17	18
65	8	8	9	10	11	12	13	14	15	17	18
60	7	8	9	10	10	11	12	14	15	16	18
55	7	8	9	9	10	11	12	13	14	16	17
50	7	8	8	9	10	11	12	13	14	16	17
45	6	7	8	9	9	10	11	12	14	15	17
40	6	7	8	8	9	10	11	12	13	15	16
35	5	6	7	8	8	9	10	12	13	14	16
30	5	6	7	7	8	9	10	12	13	14	16
25	5	5	6	7	8	9	10	11	13	14	16
20	5	5	6	6	7	8	9	11	12	13	15
15	4	4	5	6	6	7	9	10	11	13	15
10	3	3	4	4	5	6	8	9	11	13	15
5	2	2	3	4	4	5	6	8	10	12	14

Table 5.16. Fitted percentile scores for Later Gestures (CDI: Words and Gestures)—both sexes combined

%ile rank	Age (in months)										
	8	9	10	11	12	13	14	15	16	17	18
99	23	28	32	35	38	40	42	43	44	45	45
95	14	17	21	24	28	31	34	37	39	41	42
90	10	13	17	21	25	28	32	35	38	40	41
85	9	12	15	18	22	26	30	33	36	38	40
80	8	11	14	17	20	24	28	31	34	37	39
75	7	10	12	15	19	22	26	30	33	36	38
70	6	8	11	14	17	21	25	29	32	35	38
65	6	8	10	13	16	20	24	27	31	34	37
60	5	7	9	12	15	18	22	26	30	33	36
55	5	7	9	11	14	18	21	25	29	32	35
50	4	6	8	10	13	16	20	24	27	31	34
45	4	6	7	10	12	16	19	23	27	30	33
40	3	4	6	8	11	14	18	22	26	30	33
35	3	4	5	7	10	13	17	21	25	29	32
30	3	4	5	7	9	12	16	19	23	27	31
25	3	3	5	6	9	11	14	18	22	26	30
20	2	3	4	5	7	10	13	17	21	25	30
15	2	2	3	5	6	9	12	15	19	23	27
10	1	2	2	3	5	7	10	13	16	20	25
5	0	0	0	1	1	2	5	9	15	18	22

Table 5.17. Fitted percentile scores for Later Gestures (CDI: Words and Gestures)—girls

%ile rank	Age (in months)										
	8	**9**	**10**	**11**	**12**	**13**	**14**	**15**	**16**	**17**	**18**
99	21	25	30	34	37	39	41	43	44	44	45
95	13	17	21	26	30	34	37	40	42	43	44
90	10	14	17	21	25	29	33	36	39	41	42
85	9	12	15	19	23	27	31	35	38	40	42
80	8	10	14	17	21	26	30	33	36	39	41
75	7	10	13	16	20	24	28	31	35	37	40
70	6	8	11	14	18	22	26	30	34	37	39
65	6	8	10	13	17	21	25	29	33	36	38
60	5	7	9	12	16	20	24	28	32	35	38
55	4	6	8	11	14	18	22	27	31	34	37
50	4	6	8	10	13	17	21	26	30	33	36
45	3	5	7	9	12	16	20	24	28	32	36
40	3	5	6	9	11	15	19	23	27	31	35
35	3	4	6	8	11	14	18	22	26	31	34
30	3	4	5	7	10	13	17	21	26	30	33
25	2	3	4	6	9	12	16	20	25	29	33
20	2	3	4	5	7	10	14	18	22	27	31
15	2	2	3	5	6	9	12	16	20	24	29
10	1	2	2	4	5	7	10	13	17	22	26
5	1	1	1	1	2	3	6	10	15	20	25

Table 5.18. Fitted percentile scores for Later Gestures (CDI: Words and Gestures)—boys

%ile rank	Age (in months)										
	8	**9**	**10**	**11**	**12**	**13**	**14**	**15**	**16**	**17**	**18**
99	20	24	27	30	33	35	38	39	41	42	43
95	15	18	21	24	28	31	33	36	38	39	41
90	12	15	17	21	24	27	30	33	35	37	39
85	11	13	16	19	22	25	28	31	34	36	38
80	8	11	13	16	20	23	26	30	33	35	37
75	8	10	12	15	18	21	25	28	31	34	36
70	7	8	11	14	17	20	23	27	30	33	36
65	6	8	10	13	15	19	22	25	29	32	35
60	5	7	9	12	14	17	21	24	28	31	34
55	5	7	9	11	14	17	20	23	27	30	33
50	4	6	7	9	12	15	18	22	26	29	32
45	4	5	7	9	11	14	18	21	25	28	32
40	3	5	6	8	11	13	17	20	24	27	31
35	3	4	5	7	10	13	16	20	23	27	31
30	3	4	5	7	9	12	15	19	23	26	30
25	3	4	5	7	9	11	14	18	21	25	29
20	2	3	4	5	7	9	12	16	20	24	28
15	2	2	3	5	6	9	11	15	19	23	26
10	0	1	1	2	3	5	8	12	15	19	24
5	0	0	0	0	1	2	4	8	13	16	18

Table 5.19. Fitted percentile scores for Words Produced (CDI: Words and Sentences)—both sexes combined

%ile rank	Age (in months)														
	16	17	18	19	20	21	22	23	24	25	26	27	28	29	30
99	372	436	494	543	581	610	632	647	658	665	670	674	676	678	679
95	253	303	354	404	452	496	533	565	591	612	629	642	651	659	665
90	179	221	268	318	368	418	464	506	542	572	597	616	632	644	653
85	145	182	224	270	319	369	418	464	505	541	571	595	615	631	643
80	124	156	194	236	282	331	380	427	471	510	545	573	597	616	631
75	108	136	170	209	252	299	347	395	441	484	521	553	580	602	620
70	94	119	149	184	224	268	314	362	409	453	493	529	559	585	606
65	83	105	132	164	201	242	287	333	380	426	468	506	540	568	592
60	72	92	116	145	178	217	259	304	351	397	441	482	518	550	576
55	61	78	99	125	156	192	233	277	324	371	418	461	500	535	564
50	52	67	86	109	137	171	209	251	297	344	391	437	478	516	548
45	43	55	72	92	117	147	183	223	268	315	363	411	455	496	532
40	37	48	62	80	102	128	160	198	239	285	332	380	426	469	508
35	32	41	54	69	88	111	139	172	210	252	297	343	390	435	476
30	26	34	44	57	73	92	117	146	180	218	261	306	353	399	443
25	22	29	37	48	62	79	100	126	156	191	231	275	320	367	412
20	19	25	32	41	53	67	84	105	131	161	195	233	275	318	363
15	14	19	24	31	40	51	66	83	104	130	161	195	234	277	321
10	10	13	17	22	29	37	48	61	77	98	122	151	184	222	263
5	7	9	11	14	18	23	29	36	45	56	70	87	107	130	158

Table 5.20. Fitted percentile scores for Words Produced (CDI: Words and Sentences)—girls

%ile rank	Age (in months)														
	16	17	18	19	20	21	22	23	24	25	26	27	28	29	30
99	362	425	482	531	571	602	625	641	653	662	668	672	675	677	678
95	288	340	393	443	489	529	562	590	612	629	642	652	659	665	669
90	220	263	310	357	404	449	489	526	557	583	604	621	635	645	654
85	176	215	259	306	355	403	448	490	526	558	584	605	623	636	647
80	141	176	217	262	310	360	408	455	496	533	564	590	610	627	640
75	122	154	191	234	281	330	380	427	472	512	546	575	599	618	633
70	105	133	167	207	251	299	349	398	445	488	525	558	585	606	624
65	93	119	151	188	230	277	326	375	423	468	509	543	573	597	616
60	85	108	136	170	209	252	298	346	394	440	482	520	552	579	601
55	72	93	118	149	186	228	274	322	372	420	465	505	540	570	594
50	62	81	104	132	166	205	249	296	346	395	442	485	523	555	582
45	53	69	89	114	144	180	221	266	314	363	411	457	498	534	564
40	47	61	79	101	128	160	197	238	284	331	379	425	469	508	541
35	41	53	69	88	111	140	173	211	253	299	346	392	437	479	516
30	33	43	55	71	91	116	146	181	220	264	311	359	406	451	491
25	28	36	47	60	76	97	121	151	185	223	265	310	356	401	444
20	23	29	38	48	62	78	98	123	151	185	222	264	308	352	397
15	18	23	30	38	48	61	77	96	120	147	179	214	254	296	339
10	12	16	21	27	35	45	57	73	92	115	143	176	213	254	298
5	7	9	12	16	20	27	35	45	58	74	94	118	147	181	220

Table 5.21. Fitted percentile scores for Words Produced (CDI: Words and Sentences)—boys

%ile rank	Age (in months)														
	16	17	18	19	20	21	22	23	24	25	26	27	28	29	30
99	346	399	450	496	535	569	595	617	633	645	655	662	667	671	673
95	217	266	318	371	423	471	513	550	580	604	623	637	649	657	663
90	157	195	238	285	335	384	432	476	516	550	578	601	619	634	645
85	125	157	195	238	284	333	382	429	473	513	547	575	599	617	632
80	108	135	168	206	249	294	342	389	435	477	515	547	575	598	616
75	101	126	155	188	225	266	309	354	397	439	478	513	544	570	592
70	84	106	131	161	195	234	275	319	364	407	449	487	521	551	576
65	71	89	112	139	171	207	248	291	336	381	424	465	502	535	563
60	56	72	92	117	146	181	221	265	311	359	406	450	491	527	558
55	45	59	76	97	124	155	192	234	279	327	376	423	467	506	541
50	39	51	66	85	108	137	171	209	252	299	347	395	441	483	520
45	35	46	59	76	96	121	151	186	225	269	314	361	407	450	490
40	29	38	49	63	81	103	130	162	199	240	285	332	379	425	467
35	24	32	42	54	70	89	113	142	176	215	258	304	352	399	444
30	21	28	36	47	60	76	97	122	151	185	224	267	312	358	404
25	19	24	32	41	52	67	84	106	132	163	199	238	281	326	371
20	15	20	26	33	42	54	68	86	108	134	164	199	238	280	324
15	13	16	21	27	34	44	55	70	87	109	134	164	198	235	276
10	10	13	16	20	25	32	40	50	63	78	96	118	143	173	205
5	5	6	8	11	13	17	22	28	35	44	55	69	86	107	131

Table 5.22. Fitted percentile scores for Word Forms (CDI: Words and Sentences)—both sexes combined

%ile rank	Age (in months)														
	16	17	18	19	20	21	22	23	24	25	26	27	28	29	30
99	11	13	15	17	19	20	21	22	23	24	24	25	25	25	25
95	3	4	6	7	9	11	14	16	18	20	21	22	23	24	25
90	2	2	3	5	6	8	10	12	14	16	18	20	21	23	23
85	1	2	3	3	5	6	8	9	11	13	15	17	19	21	22
80	1	2	2	3	4	5	6	8	10	11	13	15	17	19	20
75	1	1	2	2	3	4	5	7	8	10	12	14	16	17	19
70	1	1	2	2	3	3	4	6	7	9	11	13	15	17	19
65	0	0	1	1	1	2	3	4	5	7	10	12	15	17	19
60	0	0	1	1	1	2	2	3	5	6	8	10	13	15	17
55	0	0	1	1	1	2	2	3	4	5	7	9	11	14	17
50	0	0	0	0	1	1	1	2	3	4	6	9	11	14	17
45	0	0	0	0	0	0	1	1	2	3	5	8	11	14	17
40	0	0	0	0	0	0	1	1	2	3	4	7	9	13	15
35	0	0	0	0	0	0	1	1	2	3	4	6	8	11	14
30	0	0	0	0	0	0	0	1	1	2	3	4	7	10	13
25	0	0	0	0	0	0	0	0	1	1	2	4	6	9	12
20	0	0	0	0	0	0	0	0	0	1	1	2	4	6	9
15	0	0	0	0	0	0	0	0	0	0	1	1	2	4	6
10	0	0	0	0	0	0	0	0	0	0	1	1	2	3	4
5	0	0	0	0	0	0	0	0	0	0	0	0	0	0	0

Table 5.23. Fitted percentile scores for Word Forms (CDI: Words and Sentences)—girls

%ile rank	Age (in months)														
	16	17	18	19	20	21	22	23	24	25	26	27	28	29	30
99	8	10	12	15	17	19	21	22	23	24	24	25	25	25	25
95	4	5	7	9	11	13	16	18	20	21	23	24	24	25	25
90	3	4	5	6	8	10	11	14	16	17	19	21	22	23	24
85	2	2	3	4	6	7	9	11	13	15	17	19	20	21	23
80	1	2	2	3	4	6	7	9	11	13	15	17	19	21	22
75	1	1	2	3	4	5	6	8	9	11	13	15	17	19	21
70	1	1	2	2	3	4	5	7	8	10	12	14	16	18	19
65	1	1	2	2	3	4	5	6	7	9	11	12	15	17	18
60	0	0	1	1	1	2	3	4	6	7	10	12	15	17	18
55	0	0	1	1	1	2	3	4	5	7	9	11	14	16	18
50	0	0	0	0	1	1	2	2	4	5	8	10	13	15	18
45	0	0	0	0	1	1	1	2	3	5	7	9	12	15	18
40	0	0	0	0	1	1	1	2	3	4	6	8	11	14	17
35	0	0	0	0	0	0	1	1	2	3	5	8	11	14	17
30	0	0	0	0	0	0	0	1	1	2	4	6	9	13	17
25	0	0	0	0	0	0	0	1	1	2	3	5	7	11	14
20	0	0	0	0	0	0	0	0	1	1	2	3	5	8	12
15	0	0	0	0	0	0	0	0	0	1	1	3	4	7	10
10	0	0	0	0	0	0	0	0	0	0	1	1	2	3	5
5	0	0	0	0	0	0	0	0	0	0	0	1	1	2	3

Table 5.24. Fitted percentile scores for Word Forms (CDI: Words and Sentences)—boys

%ile rank	Age (in months)														
	16	17	18	19	20	21	22	23	24	25	26	27	28	29	30
99	8	10	11	13	15	17	19	20	21	22	23	24	24	25	25
95	3	4	5	6	8	10	13	15	17	19	20	22	23	24	24
90	2	2	3	4	5	7	8	10	12	14	16	18	20	21	22
85	1	2	2	3	4	5	6	8	10	12	14	16	18	19	21
80	1	2	2	3	3	4	5	7	8	10	12	14	16	17	19
75	1	1	1	2	3	3	4	5	7	8	10	12	14	16	18
70	0	0	1	1	1	2	3	4	5	7	9	11	14	16	18
65	0	0	1	1	1	2	2	3	4	6	8	10	12	14	16
60	0	0	1	1	1	1	2	3	4	5	7	9	11	13	16
55	0	0	0	0	0	1	1	2	2	4	5	8	10	13	16
50	0	0	0	0	0	0	1	1	2	3	5	7	10	13	16
45	0	0	0	0	0	0	1	1	2	3	4	6	8	11	15
40	0	0	0	0	0	0	1	1	1	2	3	5	7	10	13
35	0	0	0	0	0	0	0	1	1	2	2	4	6	9	12
30	0	0	0	0	0	0	0	0	1	1	2	3	5	8	11
25	0	0	0	0	0	0	0	0	1	1	2	3	4	6	9
20	0	0	0	0	0	0	0	0	0	1	1	2	3	4	6
15	0	0	0	0	0	0	0	0	0	0	1	1	2	3	4
10	0	0	0	0	0	0	0	0	0	0	0	0	0	1	1
5	0	0	0	0	0	0	0	0	0	0	0	0	0	0	0

Table 5.25. Fitted percentile scores for Word Endings/Part 2 (CDI: Words and Sentences)—both sexes combined

%ile rank	Age (in months)														
	16	17	18	19	20	21	22	23	24	25	26	27	28	29	30
99	6	7	8	10	12	14	17	19	22	25	27	30	32	34	36
95	2	2	2	3	4	4	5	7	8	10	12	14	16	23	26
90	0	0	0	1	1	1	2	3	4	6	9	12	16	21	26
85	0	0	0	0	1	1	1	2	3	5	7	10	14	19	23
80	0	0	0	0	0	0	1	1	2	3	5	8	12	17	23
75	0	0	0	0	0	0	1	1	2	3	4	7	10	14	19
70	0	0	0	0	0	0	0	1	1	2	3	5	8	12	18
65	0	0	0	0	0	0	0	0	1	1	2	3	6	10	15
60	0	0	0	0	0	0	0	0	0	1	2	3	5	8	12
55	0	0	0	0	0	0	0	0	0	1	1	2	4	6	10
50	0	0	0	0	0	0	0	0	0	0	0	1	1	2	3
45	0	0	0	0	0	0	0	0	0	0	0	1	1	2	2
40	0	0	0	0	0	0	0	0	0	0	0	0	1	1	1
35	0	0	0	0	0	0	0	0	0	0	0	0	0	1	1
30	0	0	0	0	0	0	0	0	0	0	0	0	0	0	0
25	0	0	0	0	0	0	0	0	0	0	0	0	0	0	0
20	0	0	0	0	0	0	0	0	0	0	0	0	0	0	0
15	0	0	0	0	0	0	0	0	0	0	0	0	0	0	0
10	0	0	0	0	0	0	0	0	0	0	0	0	0	0	0
5	0	0	0	0	0	0	0	0	0	0	0	0	0	0	0

Table 5.26. Fitted percentile scores for Word Endings/Part 2 (CDI: Words and Sentences)—girls

%ile rank	Age (in months)														
	16	17	18	19	20	21	22	23	24	25	26	27	28	29	30
99	7	8	9	10	11	12	14	15	16	18	19	21	22	24	25
95	3	4	4	5	6	7	8	9	10	11	13	14	16	18	21
90	1	1	1	2	2	3	4	5	6	8	10	12	15	18	21
85	0	0	0	1	1	1	2	3	4	6	8	11	15	18	21
80	0	0	0	0	1	1	1	2	3	5	7	10	13	17	21
75	0	0	0	0	0	1	1	2	3	4	6	8	11	16	20
70	0	0	0	0	0	0	0	1	1	2	4	6	9	13	19
65	0	0	0	0	0	0	0	1	1	2	3	5	7	11	16
60	0	0	0	0	0	0	0	0	1	1	2	4	6	10	16
55	0	0	0	0	0	0	0	0	1	1	2	3	5	9	14
50	0	0	0	0	0	0	0	0	0	1	1	2	4	7	11
45	0	0	0	0	0	0	0	0	0	0	1	1	2	4	6
40	0	0	0	0	0	0	0	0	0	0	0	1	1	1	2
35	0	0	0	0	0	0	0	0	0	0	0	0	1	1	2
30	0	0	0	0	0	0	0	0	0	0	0	0	0	1	1
25	0	0	0	0	0	0	0	0	0	0	0	0	0	1	1
20	0	0	0	0	0	0	0	0	0	0	0	0	0	0	0
15	0	0	0	0	0	0	0	0	0	0	0	0	0	0	0
10	0	0	0	0	0	0	0	0	0	0	0	0	0	0	0
5	0	0	0	0	0	0	0	0	0	0	0	0	0	0	0

Table 5.27. Fitted percentile scores for Word Endings/Part 2 (CDI: Words and Sentences)—boys

%ile rank	Age (in months)														
	16	17	18	19	20	21	22	23	24	25	26	27	28	29	30
99	3	4	5	6	8	9	11	13	16	18	21	24	27	29	32
95	0	0	1	1	1	2	3	4	6	8	11	14	18	22	26
90	0	0	0	0	0	1	1	2	3	5	7	11	16	21	27
85	0	0	0	0	0	1	1	1	2	4	6	9	13	18	24
80	0	0	0	0	0	0	0	1	1	2	4	6	10	14	20
75	0	0	0	0	0	0	0	0	1	1	3	4	7	11	17
70	0	0	0	0	0	0	0	0	1	1	2	4	6	10	15
65	0	0	0	0	0	0	0	0	1	1	2	3	5	8	12
60	0	0	0	0	0	0	0	0	0	1	1	2	3	4	7
55	0	0	0	0	0	0	0	0	0	0	0	1	1	2	3
50	0	0	0	0	0	0	0	0	0	0	0	1	1	1	2
45	0	0	0	0	0	0	0	0	0	0	0	0	1	1	1
40	0	0	0	0	0	0	0	0	0	0	0	0	0	0	1
35	0	0	0	0	0	0	0	0	0	0	0	0	0	0	0
30	0	0	0	0	0	0	0	0	0	0	0	0	0	0	0
25	0	0	0	0	0	0	0	0	0	0	0	0	0	0	0
20	0	0	0	0	0	0	0	0	0	0	0	0	0	0	0
15	0	0	0	0	0	0	0	0	0	0	0	0	0	0	0
10	0	0	0	0	0	0	0	0	0	0	0	0	0	0	0
5	0	0	0	0	0	0	0	0	0	0	0	0	0	0	0

Table 5.28. Fitted percentile scores for Examples/M3L (CDI: Words and Sentences)—both sexes combined

%ile rank	Age (in months)														
	16	17	18	19	20	21	22	23	24	25	26	27	28	29	30
99	4.0	5.0	6.3	7.7	9.3	11.1	12.9	14.6	16.3	17.9	19.2	20.4	21.4	22.2	22.8
95	3.5	4.0	4.6	5.2	5.8	6.5	7.3	8.1	9.0	9.9	10.8	11.8	12.7	13.7	14.6
90	2.9	3.3	3.8	4.3	4.9	5.5	6.2	6.9	7.7	8.6	9.5	10.4	11.3	12.3	13.2
85	2.5	2.9	3.3	3.7	4.2	4.7	5.3	5.9	6.6	7.4	8.2	9.0	9.9	10.7	11.7
80	2.3	2.6	3.0	3.4	3.9	4.3	4.9	5.5	6.1	6.8	7.5	8.3	9.1	10.0	10.9
75	2.2	2.5	2.8	3.2	3.6	4.0	4.5	5.0	5.6	6.2	6.8	7.5	8.3	9.1	9.9
70	1.7	2.0	2.3	2.6	3.0	3.5	3.9	4.5	5.0	5.7	6.4	7.1	7.9	8.8	9.6
65	1.7	1.9	2.2	2.5	2.9	3.2	3.7	4.1	4.7	5.2	5.9	6.5	7.3	8.0	8.8
60	1.6	1.8	2.1	2.4	2.7	3.0	3.5	3.9	4.4	5.0	5.6	6.2	6.9	7.7	8.5
55	1.3	1.5	1.8	2.0	2.4	2.7	3.1	3.6	4.1	4.6	5.2	5.9	6.6	7.4	8.2
50	1.3	1.5	1.7	1.9	2.2	2.6	2.9	3.3	3.8	4.3	4.9	5.5	6.2	6.9	7.7
45	1.1	1.2	1.4	1.7	1.9	2.2	2.6	2.9	3.4	3.9	4.4	5.0	5.7	6.4	7.2
40	1.1	1.2	1.4	1.6	1.9	2.2	2.5	2.8	3.2	3.6	4.1	4.6	5.2	5.8	6.5
35	1.0	1.2	1.3	1.5	1.7	2.0	2.3	2.6	3.0	3.4	3.8	4.3	4.9	5.5	6.1
30	1.0	1.0	1.1	1.3	1.5	1.8	2.0	2.3	2.7	3.1	3.5	4.0	4.5	5.1	5.8
25	1.0	1.0	1.0	1.2	1.4	1.6	1.8	2.1	2.4	2.8	3.2	3.6	4.1	4.6	5.2
20	1.0	1.0	1.0	1.1	1.3	1.4	1.6	1.9	2.1	2.4	2.8	3.1	3.5	4.0	4.5
15	1.0	1.0	1.0	1.1	1.2	1.4	1.6	1.8	2.0	2.3	2.6	2.9	3.2	3.6	4.1
10	1.0	1.0	1.0	1.0	1.1	1.2	1.4	1.5	1.7	1.9	2.1	2.4	2.6	2.9	3.2
5	1.0	1.0	1.0	1.0	1.0	1.1	1.1	1.2	1.3	1.4	1.5	1.6	1.7	1.8	2.0

Key: M3L = mean length of the three longest sentences.

Table 5.29. Fitted percentile scores for Examples/M3L (CDI: Words and Sentences)—girls

%ile rank	Age (in months)														
	16	17	18	19	20	21	22	23	24	25	26	27	28	29	30
99	4.5	5.4	6.4	7.5	8.8	10.1	11.5	12.9	14.3	15.6	16.9	18.1	19.2	20.1	20.9
95	3.5	4.0	4.6	5.3	6.0	6.8	7.7	8.6	9.6	10.6	11.7	12.7	13.8	14.8	15.8
90	3.0	3.4	3.9	4.5	5.1	5.8	6.5	7.3	8.1	9.0	10.0	10.9	11.9	12.9	13.9
85	2.6	3.0	3.5	3.9	4.5	5.1	5.7	6.4	7.2	8.0	8.9	9.8	10.7	11.7	12.7
80	2.5	2.8	3.2	3.6	4.1	4.6	5.2	5.9	6.6	7.3	8.1	8.9	9.8	10.7	11.6
75	2.3	2.6	3.0	3.4	3.8	4.3	4.8	5.4	6.1	6.8	7.5	8.3	9.1	9.9	10.8
70	2.2	2.5	2.8	3.2	3.6	4.1	4.6	5.1	5.7	6.4	7.0	7.8	8.6	9.4	10.2
65	1.9	2.2	2.5	2.8	3.2	3.6	4.1	4.6	5.2	5.8	6.5	7.2	8.0	8.8	9.7
60	1.7	1.9	2.2	2.5	2.9	3.3	3.7	4.2	4.8	5.4	6.0	6.8	7.5	8.3	9.2
55	1.6	1.9	2.1	2.4	2.8	3.1	3.6	4.0	4.5	5.1	5.7	6.3	7.0	7.7	8.5
50	1.4	1.6	1.9	2.1	2.5	2.8	3.2	3.7	4.2	4.7	5.3	6.0	6.7	7.5	8.3
45	1.3	1.5	1.7	2.0	2.3	2.6	3.0	3.4	3.9	4.4	5.0	5.6	6.3	7.0	7.8
40	1.2	1.4	1.6	1.8	2.1	2.4	2.8	3.1	3.6	4.1	4.6	5.2	5.8	6.5	7.3
35	1.1	1.3	1.5	1.7	1.9	2.2	2.6	2.9	3.4	3.9	4.4	5.0	5.6	6.3	7.1
30	1.0	1.1	1.2	1.4	1.7	1.9	2.2	2.6	3.0	3.4	3.9	4.5	5.1	5.8	6.5
25	1.0	1.0	1.1	1.2	1.5	1.7	2.0	2.3	2.6	3.0	3.5	4.0	4.5	5.2	5.9
20	1.0	1.0	1.0	1.2	1.3	1.5	1.8	2.1	2.4	2.7	3.1	3.6	4.1	4.6	5.2
15	1.0	1.0	1.0	1.0	1.2	1.4	1.6	1.8	2.1	2.4	2.7	3.1	3.5	4.0	4.5
10	1.0	1.0	1.0	1.0	1.1	1.3	1.4	1.6	1.8	2.0	2.3	2.5	2.8	3.2	3.5
5	1.0	1.0	1.0	1.0	1.1	1.2	1.3	1.4	1.6	1.7	1.9	2.0	2.2	2.4	2.7

Key: M3L = mean length of the three longest sentences.

Table 5.30. Fitted percentile scores for Examples/M3L(CDI: Words and Sentences)—boys

%ile rank	Age (in months)														
	16	17	18	19	20	21	22	23	24	25	26	27	28	29	30
99	3.4	4.2	5.1	6.2	7.4	8.7	10.2	11.7	13.2	14.7	16.2	17.5	18.7	19.8	20.7
95	3.5	4.0	4.6	5.2	5.8	6.5	7.3	8.1	9.0	9.8	10.8	11.7	12.7	13.6	14.6
90	3.0	3.4	3.8	4.2	4.7	5.3	5.9	6.5	7.2	7.9	8.7	9.4	10.3	11.1	11.9
85	2.5	2.8	3.2	3.6	4.0	4.5	5.1	5.6	6.3	7.0	7.7	8.4	9.2	10.1	10.9
80	2.1	2.4	2.7	3.0	3.4	3.8	4.3	4.8	5.3	5.9	6.5	7.2	7.9	8.6	9.4
75	1.8	2.0	2.3	2.6	3.0	3.4	3.8	4.3	4.9	5.4	6.1	6.8	7.5	8.3	9.1
70	1.7	1.9	2.2	2.5	2.8	3.2	3.6	4.1	4.6	5.1	5.7	6.4	7.1	7.8	8.6
65	1.4	1.6	1.9	2.1	2.5	2.8	3.2	3.7	4.2	4.8	5.4	6.1	6.8	7.6	8.4
60	1.4	1.6	1.8	2.1	2.3	2.7	3.0	3.4	3.8	4.3	4.9	5.4	6.1	6.7	7.5
55	1.1	1.3	1.5	1.7	2.0	2.3	2.7	3.1	3.5	4.0	4.6	5.2	5.8	6.5	7.3
50	1.1	1.3	1.5	1.7	1.9	2.2	2.5	2.9	3.3	3.7	4.2	4.8	5.4	6.1	6.8
45	1.0	1.1	1.3	1.5	1.8	2.0	2.3	2.7	3.1	3.5	4.0	4.6	5.2	5.8	6.6
40	1.0	1.1	1.3	1.5	1.7	1.9	2.2	2.5	2.9	3.3	3.7	4.2	4.7	5.3	6.0
35	1.0	1.1	1.2	1.4	1.6	1.8	2.1	2.4	2.7	3.1	3.5	3.9	4.4	5.0	5.6
30	1.0	1.0	1.1	1.2	1.4	1.6	1.8	2.1	2.4	2.7	3.1	3.5	3.9	4.4	5.0
25	1.0	1.0	1.0	1.1	1.3	1.5	1.7	1.9	2.2	2.5	2.8	3.2	3.6	4.1	4.6
20	1.0	1.0	1.0	1.1	1.2	1.4	1.6	1.8	2.0	2.3	2.6	2.9	3.2	3.6	4.1
15	1.0	1.0	1.0	1.0	1.2	1.3	1.5	1.6	1.8	2.0	2.3	2.5	2.8	3.1	3.5
10	1.0	1.0	1.0	1.0	1.1	1.1	1.2	1.3	1.4	1.6	1.7	1.8	2.0	2.1	2.3
5	1.0	1.0	1.0	1.0	1.0	1.1	1.1	1.2	1.3	1.3	1.4	1.5	1.6	1.7	1.8

Key: M3L = mean length of the three longest sentences.

Table 5.31. Fitted percentile scores for Complexity (CDI: Words and Sentences)—both sexes combined

%ile rank	Age (in months)														
	16	17	18	19	20	21	22	23	24	25	26	27	28	29	30
99	14	18	21	24	27	30	32	34	35	36	36	37	37	37	37
95	4	5	8	11	15	20	24	28	31	34	35	36	37	37	37
90	1	1	2	3	5	8	13	18	24	29	32	35	36	37	37
85	0	0	1	1	2	4	6	11	17	23	28	32	35	36	37
80	0	0	0	1	1	3	5	8	13	19	26	30	34	36	37
75	0	0	0	0	1	1	3	5	9	15	22	28	32	35	36
70	0	0	0	0	1	1	2	4	8	13	19	26	31	34	36
65	0	0	0	0	0	1	2	3	6	11	17	23	29	33	35
60	0	0	0	0	0	1	1	3	5	9	15	21	27	31	34
55	0	0	0	0	0	0	1	2	4	7	11	18	24	30	33
50	0	0	0	0	0	0	1	1	2	5	9	15	22	28	33
45	0	0	0	0	0	0	0	1	2	4	7	12	19	26	31
40	0	0	0	0	0	0	0	1	1	3	5	9	15	22	28
35	0	0	0	0	0	0	0	0	1	2	4	7	12	18	25
30	0	0	0	0	0	0	0	0	1	1	2	4	8	13	19
25	0	0	0	0	0	0	0	0	0	1	2	3	5	9	14
20	0	0	0	0	0	0	0	0	0	0	1	1	3	4	7
15	0	0	0	0	0	0	0	0	0	0	0	1	1	1	2
10	0	0	0	0	0	0	0	0	0	0	0	0	0	0	0
5	0	0	0	0	0	0	0	0	0	0	0	0	0	0	0

Table 5.32. Fitted percentile scores for Complexity (CDI: Words and Sentences)—girls

%ile rank	Age (in months)														
	16	17	18	19	20	21	22	23	24	25	26	27	28	29	30
99	12	15	18	22	26	29	31	33	35	36	36	37	37	37	37
95	4	6	9	12	17	21	26	29	32	34	35	36	37	37	37
90	1	1	2	4	6	10	16	22	27	31	34	36	37	37	37
85	0	1	1	3	5	8	12	17	23	28	32	34	36	37	37
80	0	1	1	2	3	5	9	14	19	25	30	33	35	36	37
75	0	0	0	1	2	3	5	9	15	21	27	31	34	36	37
70	0	0	0	0	1	1	3	6	10	16	23	29	33	36	37
65	0	0	0	0	1	1	2	5	8	14	20	27	31	34	36
60	0	0	0	0	0	1	2	4	7	12	18	25	30	34	36
55	0	0	0	0	0	1	1	2	5	9	14	21	28	32	35
50	0	0	0	0	0	0	1	2	4	7	13	19	26	31	34
45	0	0	0	0	0	0	1	2	3	6	11	17	24	30	33
40	0	0	0	0	0	0	1	1	2	5	9	15	22	29	33
35	0	0	0	0	0	0	0	1	1	3	6	11	18	25	31
30	0	0	0	0	0	0	0	0	1	2	4	8	14	21	28
25	0	0	0	0	0	0	0	0	1	1	3	5	9	15	22
20	0	0	0	0	0	0	0	0	0	1	1	2	4	7	12
15	0	0	0	0	0	0	0	0	0	0	1	1	2	4	7
10	0	0	0	0	0	0	0	0	0	0	0	0	1	1	2
5	0	0	0	0	0	0	0	0	0	0	0	0	0	0	0

Table 5.33.   Fitted percentile scores for Complexity (CDI: Words and Sentences)—boys

%ile rank	Age (in months)														
	16	17	18	19	20	21	22	23	24	25	26	27	28	29	30
99	12	15	18	22	25	28	31	33	34	35	36	37	37	37	37
95	4	5	8	11	14	18	22	26	29	31	33	35	36	37	37
90	1	1	2	3	4	7	10	14	19	24	28	31	34	35	36
85	0	0	0	1	1	3	5	8	13	19	25	30	33	35	36
80	0	0	0	0	1	1	2	5	8	14	20	26	31	34	36
75	0	0	0	0	1	1	2	4	7	11	17	24	29	33	35
70	0	0	0	0	0	1	2	3	5	9	15	21	27	31	34
65	0	0	0	0	0	1	1	2	4	8	12	18	24	29	33
60	0	0	0	0	0	0	1	2	3	6	10	16	22	28	33
55	0	0	0	0	0	0	0	1	2	4	7	12	18	25	30
50	0	0	0	0	0	0	0	1	2	3	6	10	16	23	29
45	0	0	0	0	0	0	0	1	1	2	4	7	13	19	26
40	0	0	0	0	0	0	0	0	1	2	3	6	10	15	22
35	0	0	0	0	0	0	0	0	0	1	2	3	6	10	16
30	0	0	0	0	0	0	0	0	0	1	1	3	5	8	13
25	0	0	0	0	0	0	0	0	0	0	1	1	2	3	5
20	0	0	0	0	0	0	0	0	0	0	0	1	1	2	3
15	0	0	0	0	0	0	0	0	0	0	0	0	0	1	1
10	0	0	0	0	0	0	0	0	0	0	0	0	0	0	0
5	0	0	0	0	0	0	0	0	0	0	0	0	0	0	0

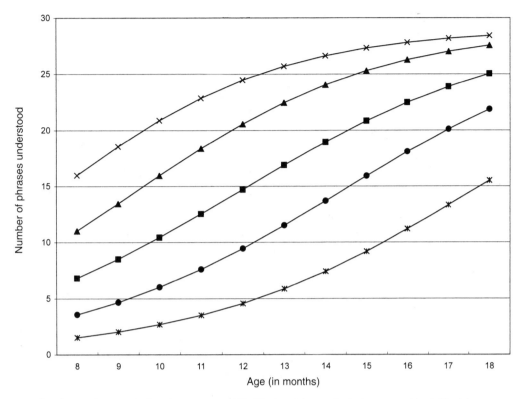

Figure 5.1. Fitted percentile scores for Phrases Understood (CDI: Words and Gestures)—both sexes combined. (*Key:* ✕ = 90th percentile; ▲ = 75th percentile; ■ = 50th percentile; ● = 25th percentile; ✸ = 10th percentile.)

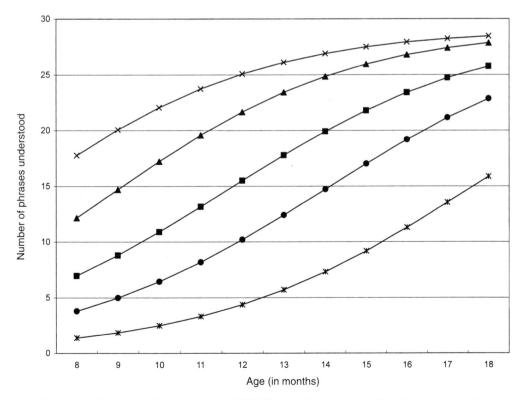

Figure 5.2. Fitted percentile scores for Phrases Understood (CDI: Words and Gestures)—girls. (*Key:* ✕ = 90th percentile; ▲ = 75th percentile; ■ = 50th percentile; ● = 25th percentile; ✸ = 10th percentile.)

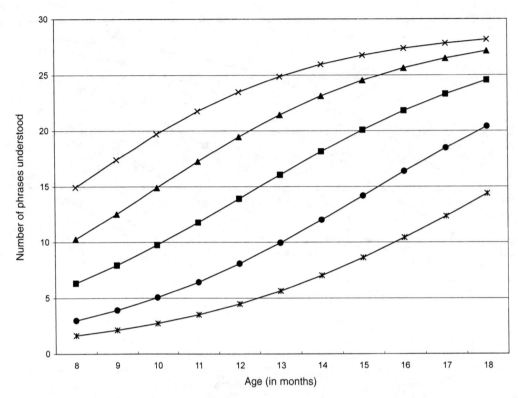

Figure 5.3. Fitted percentile scores for Phrases Understood (CDI: Words and Gestures)—boys. (*Key:* ✕ = 90th percentile; ▲ = 75th percentile; ■ = 50th percentile; ● = 25th percentile; ✳ = 10th percentile.)

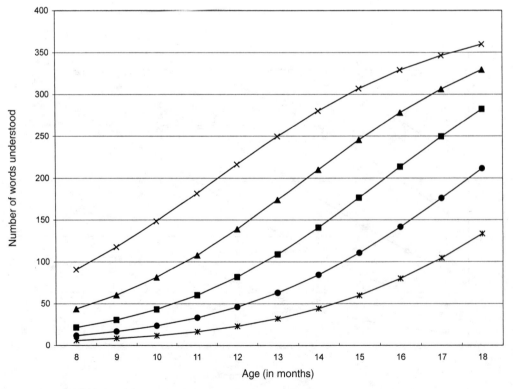

Figure 5.4. Fitted percentile scores for Words Understood (CDI: Words and Gestures)—both sexes combined. (*Key:* ✕ = 90th percentile; ▲ = 75th percentile; ■ = 50th percentile; ● = 25th percentile; ✳ = 10th percentile.)

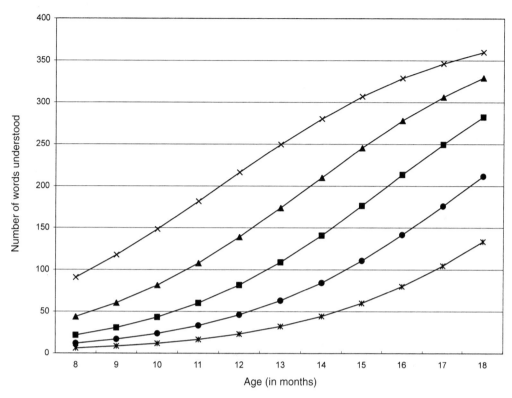

Figure 5.5. Fitted percentile scores for Words Understood (CDI: Words and Gestures)—girls. (*Key:* = ✕ 90th percentile; ▲ = 75th percentile; ■ = 50th percentile; ● = 25th percentile; ✳ = 10th percentile.)

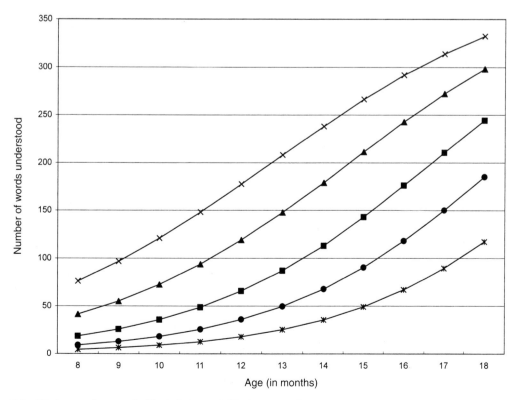

Figure 5.6. Fitted percentile scores for Words Understood (CDI: Words and Gestures)—boys. (*Key:* ✕ = 90th percentile; ▲ = 75th percentile; ■ = 50th percentile; ● = 25th percentile; ✳ = 10th percentile.)

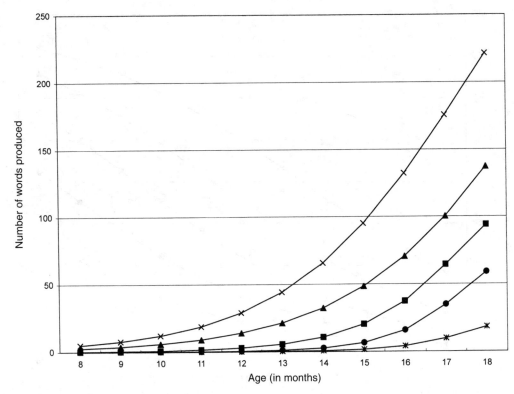

Figure 5.7. Fitted percentile scores for Words Produced (CDI: Words and Gestures)—both sexes combined. (*Key:* ✕ = 90th percentile; ▲ = 75th percentile; ■ = 50th percentile; ● = 25th percentile; ✳ = 10th percentile.)

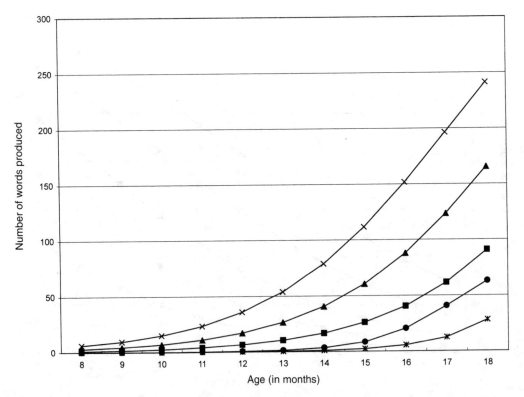

Figure 5.8. Fitted percentile scores for Words Produced (CDI: Words and Gestures)—girls. (*Key:* ✕ = 90th percentile; ▲ = 75th percentile; ■ = 50th percentile; ● = 25th percentile; ✳ = 10th percentile.)

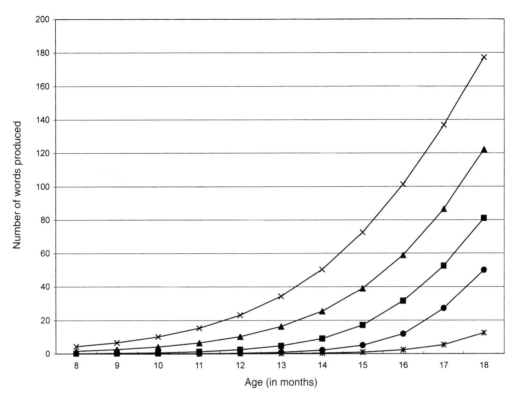

Figure 5.9. Fitted percentile scores for Words Produced (CDI: Words and Gestures)—boys. (*Key:* ✕ = 90th percentile; ▲ = 75th percentile; ■ = 50th percentile; ● = 25th percentile; ✳ = 10th percentile.)

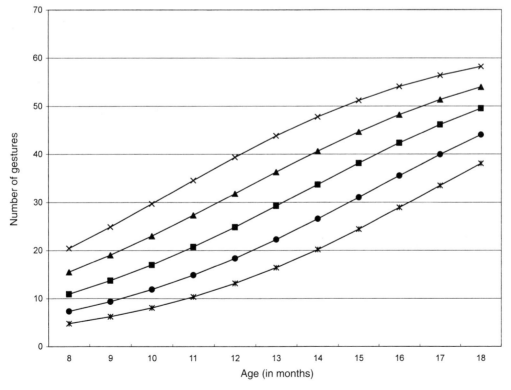

Figure 5.10. Fitted percentile scores for Total Gestures (CDI: Words and Gestures)—both sexes combined. (*Key:* ✕ = 90th percentile; ▲ = 75th percentile; ■ = 50th percentile; ● = 25th percentile; ✳ = 10th percentile.)

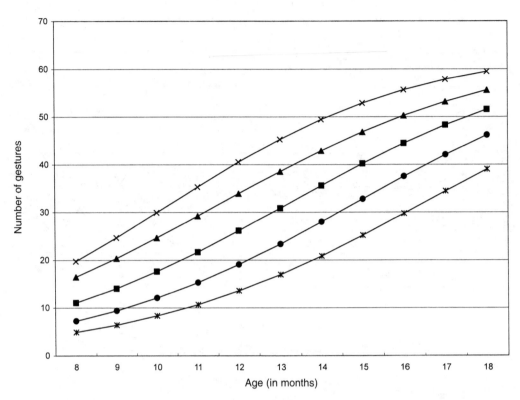

Figure 5.11. Fitted percentile scores for Total Gestures (CDI: Words and Gestures)—girls. (*Key:* ✕ = 90th percentile; ▲ = 75th percentile; ■ = 50th percentile; ● = 25th percentile; ✳ = 10th percentile.)

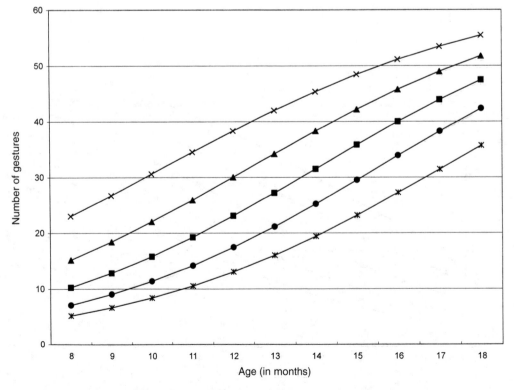

Figure 5.12. Fitted percentile scores for Total Gestures (CDI: Words and Gestures)—boys. (*Key:* ✕ = 90th percentile; ▲ = 75th percentile; ■ = 50th percentile; ● = 25th percentile; ✳ = 10th percentile.)

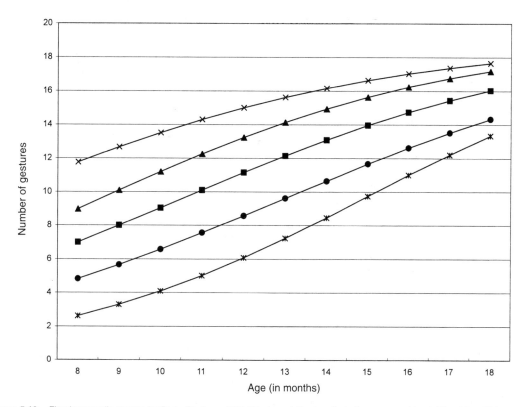

Figure 5.13. Fitted percentile scores for Early Gestures (CDI: Words and Gestures)—both sexes combined. (*Key:* ✕ = 90th percentile; ▲ = 75th percentile; ■ = 50th percentile; ● = 25th percentile; ✳ = 10th percentile.)

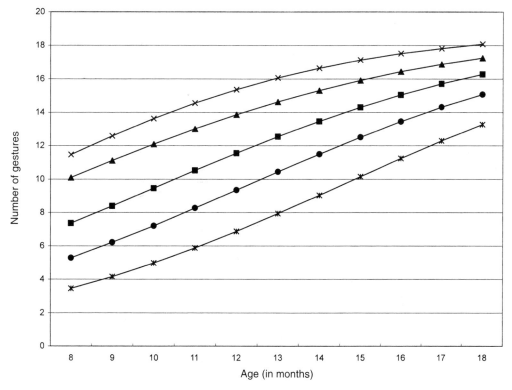

Figure 5.14. Fitted percentile scores for Early Gestures (CDI: Words and Gestures)—girls. (*Key:* ✕ = 90th percentile; ▲ = 75th percentile; ■ = 50th percentile; ● = 25th percentile; ✳ = 10th percentile.)

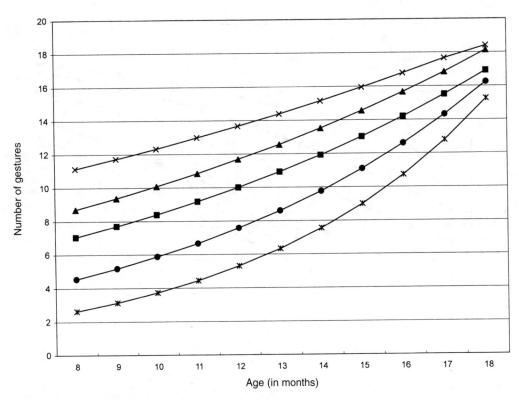

Figure 5.15. Fitted percentile scores for Early Gestures (CDI: Words and Gestures)—boys. (*Key:* ✕ = 90th percentile; ▲ = 75th percentile; ■ = 50th percentile; ● = 25th percentile; ✻ = 10th percentile.)

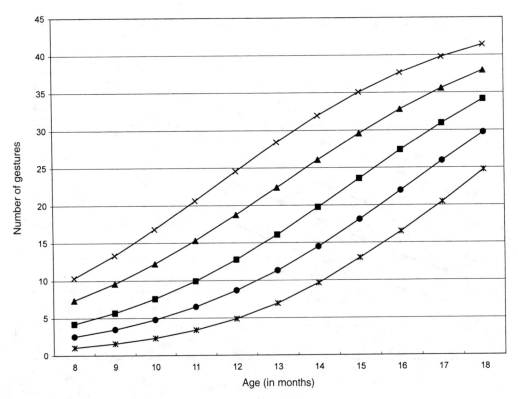

Figure 5.16. Fitted percentile scores for Later Gestures (CDI: Words and Gestures)—both sexes combined. (*Key:* ✕ = 90th percentile; ▲ = 75th percentile; ■ = 50th percentile; ● = 25th percentile; ✻ = 10th percentile.)

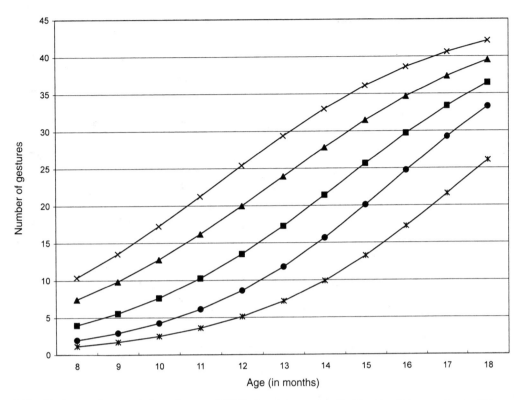

Figure 5.17. Fitted percentile scores for Later Gestures (CDI: Words and Gestures)—girls. (*Key:* ✕ = 90th percentile; ▲ = 75th percentile; ■ = 50th percentile; ● = 25th percentile; ✳ = 10th percentile.)

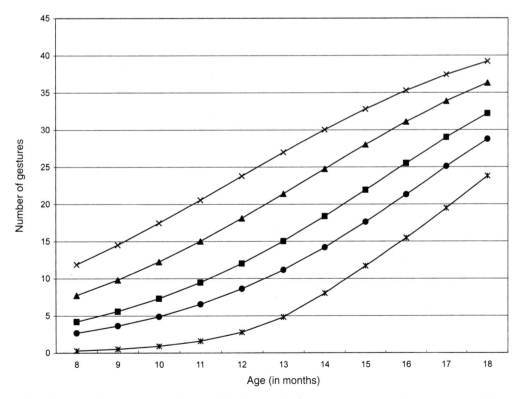

Figure 5.18. Fitted percentile scores for Later Gestures (CDI: Words and Gestures)—boys. (*Key:* ✕ = 90th percentile; ▲ = 75th percentile; ■ = 50th percentile; ● = 25th percentile; ✳ = 10th percentile.)

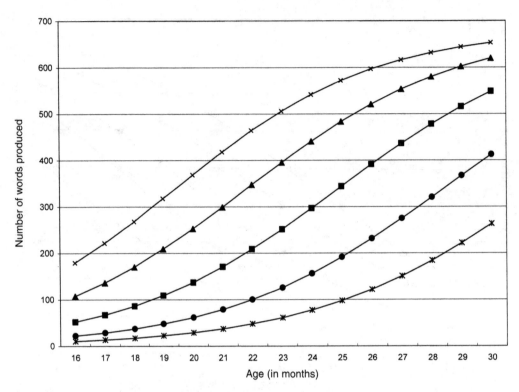

Figure 5.19. Fitted percentile scores for Words Produced (CDI: Words and Sentences)—both sexes combined. (*Key:* ✕ = 90th percentile; ▲ = 75th percentile; ■ = 50th percentile; ● = 25th percentile; ✳ = 10th percentile.)

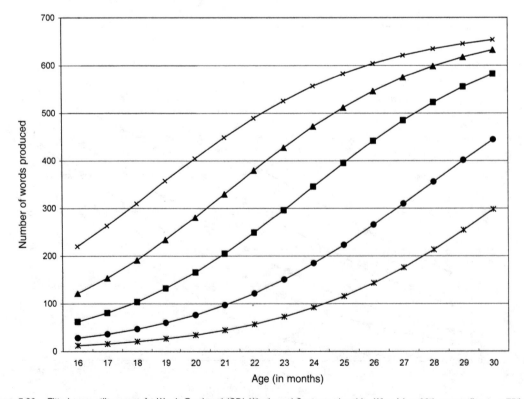

Figure 5.20. Fitted percentile scores for Words Produced (CDI: Words and Sentences)—girls. (*Key:* ✕ = 90th percentile; ▲ = 75th percentile; ■ = 50th percentile; ● = 25th percentile; ✳ = 10th percentile.)

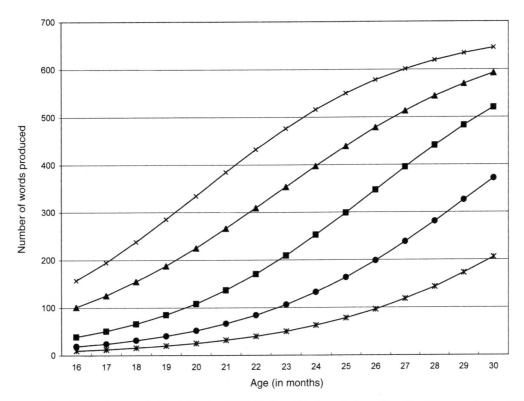

Figure 5.21. Fitted percentile scores for Words Produced (CDI: Words and Sentences)—boys. (*Key:* ✕ = 90th percentile; ▲ = 75th percentile; ■ = 50th percentile; ● = 25th percentile; ✳ = 10th percentile.)

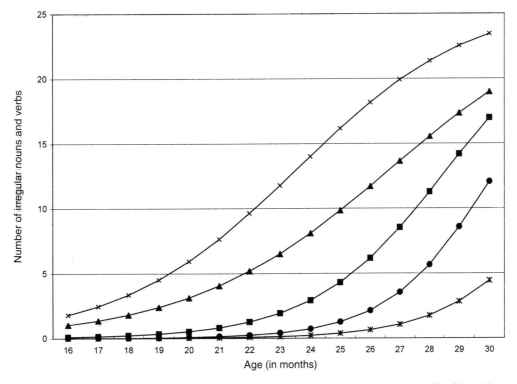

Figure 5.22. Fitted percentile scores for Word Forms (CDI: Words and Sentences)—both sexes combined. (*Key:* ✕ = 90th percentile; ▲ = 75th percentile; ■ = 50th percentile; ● = 25th percentile; ✳ = 10th percentile.)

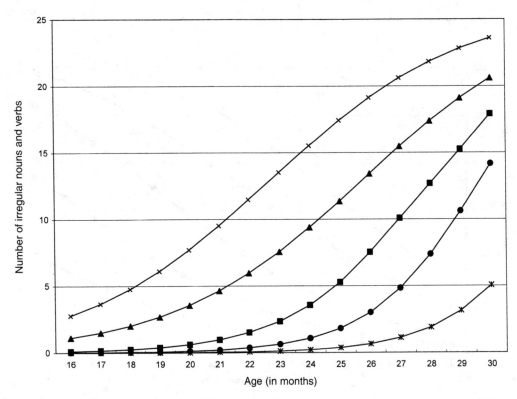

Figure 5.23. Fitted percentile scores for Word Forms (CDI: Words and Sentences)—girls. (*Key:* ✕ = 90th percentile; ▲ = 75th percentile; ■ = 50th percentile; ● = 25th percentile; ✶ = 10th percentile.)

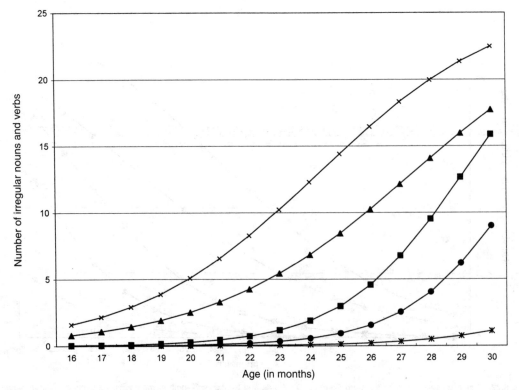

Figure 5.24. Fitted percentile scores for Word Forms (CDI: Words and Sentences)—boys. (*Key:* ✕ = 90th percentile; ▲ = 75th percentile; ■ = 50th percentile; ● = 25th percentile; ✶ = 10th percentile.)

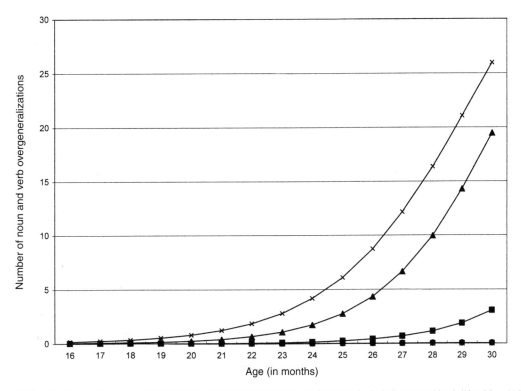

Figure 5.25. Fitted percentile scores for Word Endings/Part 2 (CDI: Words and Sentences)—both sexes combined. (*Key:* ✕ = 90th percentile; ▲ = 75th percentile; ■ = 50th percentile; ● = 25th percentile; ✳ = 10th percentile.)

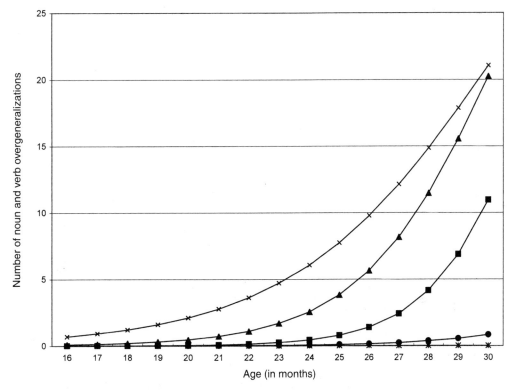

Figure 5.26. Fitted percentile scores for Word Endings/Part 2 (CDI: Words and Sentences)—girls. (*Key:* ✕ = 90th percentile; ▲ = 75th percentile; ■ = 50th percentile; ● = 25th percentile; ✳ = 10th percentile.)

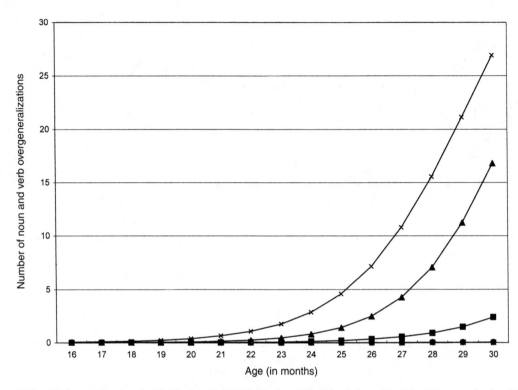

Figure 5.27. Fitted percentile scores for Word Endings/Part 2 (CDI: Words and Sentences)—boys. (*Key:* ✕ = 90th percentile; ▲ = 75th percentile; ■ = 50th percentile; ● = 25th percentile; ✳ = 10th percentile.)

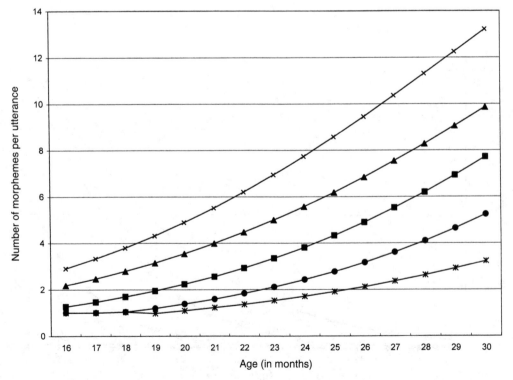

Figure 5.28. Fitted percentile scores for Examples/mean length of the three longest sentences (M3L) (CDI: Words and Sentences)—both sexes combined. (*Key:* ✕ = 90th percentile; ▲ = 75th percentile; ■ = 50th percentile; ● = 25th percentile; ✳ = 10th percentile; M3L = mean length of the three longest sentences.)

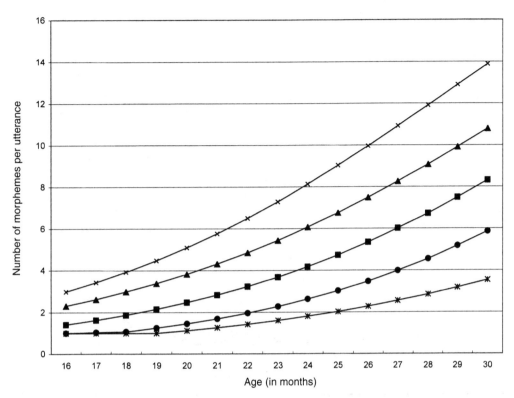

Figure 5.29. Fitted percentile scores for Examples/mean length of the three longest sentences (M3L) (CDI: Words and Sentences)—girls. (*Key:* ✕ = 90th percentile; ▲ = 75th percentile; ■ = 50th percentile; ● = 25th percentile; ✻ = 10th percentile; M3L = mean length of the three longest sentences.)

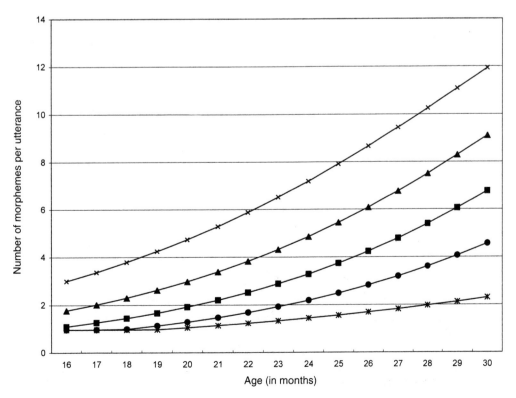

Figure 5.30. Fitted percentile scores for Examples/mean length of the three longest sentences (M3L) (CDI: Words and Sentences)—boys. (*Key:* ✕ = 90th percentile; ▲ = 75th percentile; ■ = 50th percentile; ● = 25th percentile; ✻ = 10th percentile; M3L = mean length of the three longest sentences.)

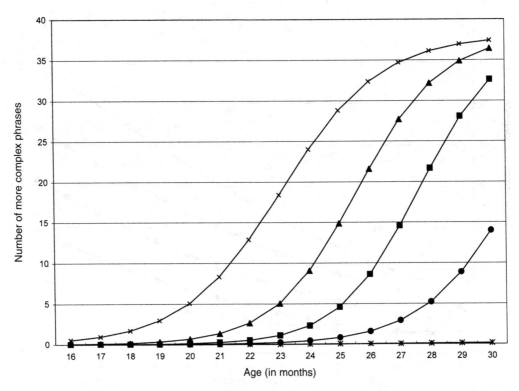

Figure 5.31. Fitted percentile scores for Complexity (CDI: Words and Sentences)—both sexes combined. (*Key:* ✕ = 90th percentile; ▲ = 75th percentile; ■ = 50th percentile; ● = 25th percentile; ✖ = 10th percentile.)

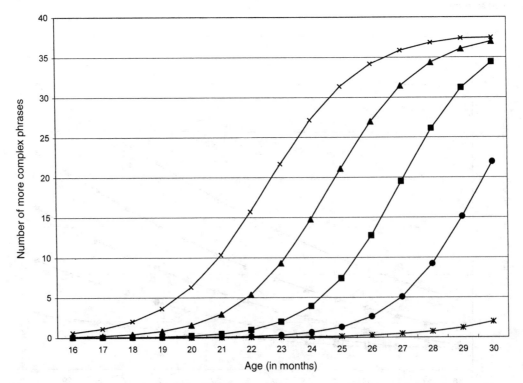

Figure 5.32. Fitted percentile scores for Complexity (CDI: Words and Sentences)—girls. (*Key:* ✕ = 90th percentile; ▲ = 75th percentile; ■ = 50th percentile; ● = 25th percentile; ✖ = 10th percentile.)

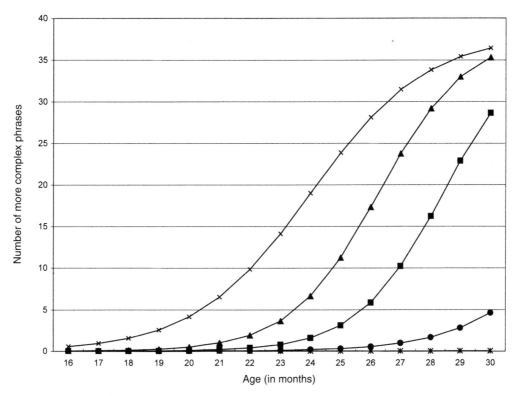

Figure 5.33. Fitted percentile scores for Complexity (CDI: Words and Sentences)—boys. (*Key:* ✕ = 90th percentile; ▲ = 75th percentile; ■ = 50th percentile; ● = 25th percentile; ✳ = 10th percentile.)

6

THE MACARTHUR-BATES COMMUNICATIVE DEVELOPMENT INVENTORY-III

The MacArthur-Bates Communicative Development Inventories have proven to be reliable, valid, and highly useful measures of language and communicative development for 8- to 30-month old typically developing children and older children in this developmental range. Their success, along with the fact that reliable and valid variance remained at 30 months for the CDI: Words and Sentences, suggested that an upward extension for 3-year-olds might be both useful and feasible. This age is often a focus in both research and clinical work. In research, measures at age 3 become considerably more valid as predictors of abilities in later childhood and hence are especially appropriate for measuring the consequences of early experiences, such as preterm birth, ear infections, poverty, type of child care, and intervention programs. In clinical work, the Individuals with Disabilities Education Improvement Act of 2004 (PL 108-446, or "IDEA 2004") mandates that schools provide appropriate services for children between 3 and 5 years of age with developmental delays; thus, the need for effective tools for evaluation at age 3 or shortly thereafter has increased. The MacArthur-Bates Communicative Development Inventory–III (CDI-III) has been developed to serve this function. The name "CDI-III" reflects its developmental potential. It is the third in the CDI series, which began with the CDI: Words and Gestures and the CDI: Words and Sentences. In addition, it was specifically designed for use with 3-year-olds.

COMPONENTS OF THE CDI-III

The CDI: Words and Gestures and the CDI: Words and Sentences each include an extensive vocabulary checklist. After the age of 30 months, it is impractical to devise a list of words that is even approximately comprehensive. Only a systematic sampling is possible. The CDI-III is a brief measure, printed on the front and back of a single page.

Vocabulary Checklist

The first component is a 100-item vocabulary checklist. Individual item norms for the Vocabulary Checklist component of the CDI: Words and Sentences form (Dale & Fenson, 1996) were reviewed to select items of appropriate difficulty. Two rounds of pilot testing revealed that ceiling effects were reached for many words not long after children were 30 months of age, meaning that the measure required new words. The final list of 100 words includes 45 words from the CDI: Words and Sentences form and 55 new words, which were drawn from a variety of tests and the child language research literature. This component yields a score ranging from 0 to 100.

Sentences

The second component consists of 13 questions about the child's word combinations. The first question on the CDI: Words and Sentences form also found whether the child is combining words yet. There are three alternative responses: *not yet, sometimes,* and *often.* If the response is *not yet,* the parent is finished completing the form. If the parent selects *sometimes* or *often,* he or she moves on to the next section. There are 12 sentence pairs, each of which has a related meaning but differs in grammatical level, similar to the 37 sentence pairs in the Complexity section of the CDI: Words and Sentences form. In each case, the first sentence has a developmentally simpler form. The directions ask the parent to indicate the sentence in each pair "that sounds MOST like the way your child talks at the moment. If your child is saying sentences even more complicated than the two provided, mark the second one." The set of 12 sentence pairs includes five drawn from the CDI: Words and Sentences form and seven new items developed to reach the appropriate difficulty level. As was the case for the CDI-III vocabulary measure, the development of this 12-item list was based on a review of the literature and tested in a pilot study. This component yields a score that is the total number of sentence pairs for which the parent checked the second, more complex sentence. The maximum score is 12. Note that a 0 is received both by children who are not combining words and by children who are combining words but in every case are still using the developmentally simpler form.

Using Language

The third and final component consists of 12 yes-or-no questions about the child's language use. These include questions about comprehension (e.g., "Does your child know his/her right hand from his/her left hand?"), semantics (e.g., "Does your child ever ask what a particular word means?"), and syntax (e.g., "Does your child give reasons for things, using the word 'because'?"). These items were developed on the basis of a literature review of tests and questionnaires and tested in a pilot study. This component yields a score that is the total number of *yes* answers, and scores range from 0 to 12.

THE NORMING STUDY

Families who were available through a university subject pool database were sent letters at the appropriate ages. Additional data for children at 36 months were obtained from an ongoing study in the San Diego, California, area. Examination of the results determined that despite repeated revisions to make the instrument more difficult, there appeared to be some ceiling effects after 37 months of age. As a result, the norming was confined to the 30- to 37-month age range, with 2-month age windows. Table 6.1 describes the resulting norming sample with respect to age and gender.

Table 6.1. Composition of the norming sample for the MacArthur-Bates Communicative Development Inventory–III (CDI-III)

Age in months	Gender		Total
	Male	Female	
30–31	43	34	77
32–33	38	29	67
34–35	35	27	62
36–37	71	79	150
Total	187	169	356

Maternal education level was available for only 169 children (47.5% of the sample). Because this initial norming was done primarily with families who had volunteered for research, it skewed rather substantially toward parents with high educational level. The four maternal education categories of Table 4.3 (some high school or less, high school diploma, some college education, and college diploma) were used and resulted in percentages of .6, 9.5, 20.1, and 69.8, respectively. These figures diverge significantly from U.S. census norms. For this reason, at the present time the applicability of norms derived from this sample for children from families with low incomes and/or education levels is unknown.

DEVELOPMENTAL TRENDS, NORMS, AND SEX DIFFERENCES

All three measures showed developmental increase across the 30- to 37-month age range, substantial variation at each age, and modest but significant sex differences favoring girls. Figures 6.1 and 6.2 illustrate this pattern for the Vocabulary Checklist measure. An analysis of variance was performed with age and sex as independent variables. Age was, as expected, highly significant as a predictor, accounting for (partial eta-squared) 18.9%, 16.5%, and 21.1% of the variance in Vocabulary Checklist, Sentences, and Using Language, respectively. Sex was also a statistically significant predictor, accounting for 2.4% of the variance in Vocabulary Checklist, 2.3% for Sentences, and 5.4% for Using Language. None of the age by sex interaction terms were significant.

Tables 6.2 through 6.10 provide percentile equivalents for the raw scores on these measures. Separate tables are provided for girls and boys, as well as a set for both sexes combined. These tables are based on a curve-fitting procedure

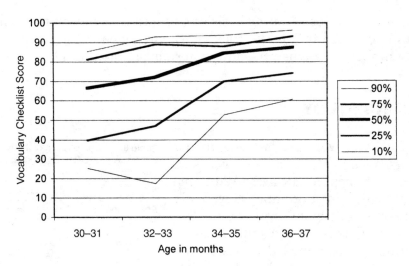

Figure 6.1. Growth in vocabulary scores for girls. (*Note:* These scores should not be interpreted as the child's total vocabulary, as only a small sample of words occur on the CDI-III.)

similar to that done for the CDI: Words and Gestures form and the CDI: Words and Sentences form.

VALIDITY OF THE CDI-III

Four studies provide concurrent validity estimates for the CDI-III. In the first, conducted by Thal (personal communication), CDI-III Vocabulary Checklist scores were compared with test scores on the Preschool Language Scale, Third Edition (PLS-3; Zimmerman, Steiner, & Pond, 1992) for a sample of 19 typically

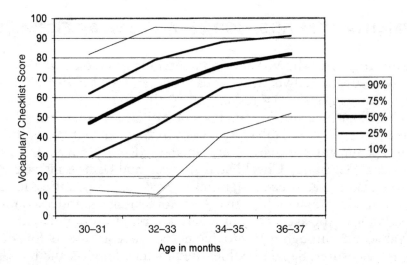

Figure 6.2. Growth in vocabulary scores for boys. (*Note:* These scores should not be interpreted as the child's total vocabulary, as only a small sample of words occur on the CDI-III.)

Table 6.2. The MacArthur-Bates Communicative Development Inventory–III (CDI-III) fitted percentile values for Vocabulary Checklist—both sexes combined

%ile rank	Age (in months)			
	30–31	32–33	34–35	36–37
99	95	98	99	100
95	91	94	96	98
90	88	92	94	96
85	86	90	93	95
80	82	87	91	94
75	78	84	89	92
70	74	81	87	91
65	69	78	86	91
60	65	75	83	89
55	62	71	81	88
50	59	70	79	86
45	54	65	75	83
40	49	61	72	81
35	46	58	69	79
30	43	55	66	76
25	38	50	62	73
20	32	44	57	69
15	25	37	50	64
10	17	28	43	59
5	10	18	29	45

Table 6.3. The MacArthur-Bates Communicative Development Inventory–III (CDI-III) fitted percentile values for Vocabulary Checklist—girls

%ile rank	Age (in months)			
	30–31	32–33	34–35	36–37
99	95	97	99	100
95	93	96	97	99
90	89	92	95	97
85	87	90	93	95
80	84	88	92	94
75	82	87	90	93
70	80	85	89	92
65	79	84	88	91
60	76	82	87	90
55	73	80	85	90
50	67	75	82	87
45	65	73	80	86
40	63	70	77	83
35	54	64	72	79
30	49	60	69	77
25	44	55	65	74
20	37	47	58	68
15	28	40	52	65
10	21	32	46	60
5	12	20	33	48

Table 6.4. The MacArthur-Bates Communicative Development Inventory–III (CDI-III) fitted percentile values for Vocabulary Checklist—boys

%ile rank	Age (in months)			
	30–31	32–33	34–35	36–37
99	94	97	99	100
95	92	95	97	98
90	89	92	94	96
85	84	88	92	95
80	75	84	90	94
75	69	79	87	92
70	63	75	84	91
65	61	72	82	88
60	60	71	80	87
55	57	68	78	85
50	51	63	74	83
45	49	61	72	81
40	46	58	70	79
35	43	55	66	76
30	40	52	64	74
25	34	47	60	72
20	27	40	54	68
15	22	34	48	62
10	14	24	38	55
5	0	2	9	30

Table 6.5. The MacArthur-Bates Communicative Development Inventory–III (CDI-III) fitted percentile values for Sentences—both sexes combined

%ile rank	Age (in months)			
	30–31	32–33	34–35	36–37
99	12	12	12	12
95	12	12	12	12
90	12	12	12	12
85	12	12	12	12
80	11	12	12	12
75	10	11	12	12
70	10	11	12	12
65	9	10	12	12
60	9	10	12	12
55	8	10	11	12
50	7	9	11	12
45	7	9	10	11
40	6	8	10	11
35	5	7	9	10
30	5	6	8	10
25	4	6	7	9
20	2	4	7	9
15	1	3	6	9
10	1	2	3	7
5	0	0	1	5

Table 6.6. The MacArthur-Bates Communicative Development Inventory–III (CDI-III) fitted percentile values for Sentences—girls

%ile rank	Age (in months)			
	30–31	32–33	34–35	36–37
99	12	12	12	12
95	12	12	12	12
90	12	12	12	12
85	12	12	12	12
80	12	12	12	12
75	11	12	12	12
70	11	11	12	12
65	10	11	12	12
60	10	11	12	12
55	10	11	12	12
50	9	10	11	12
45	8	10	11	12
40	7	9	11	12
35	6	8	10	11
30	6	8	10	11
25	5	7	9	10
20	4	6	8	10
15	3	5	7	9
10	0	0	2	5
5	0	0	0	1

Table 6.7. The MacArthur-Bates Communicative Development Inventory–III (CDI-III) fitted percentile values for Sentences—boys

%ile rank	Age (in months)			
	30–31	32–33	34–35	36–37
99	12	12	12	12
95	12	12	12	12
90	12	12	12	12
85	11	11	12	12
80	10	11	12	12
75	9	11	12	12
70	9	10	12	12
65	8	10	11	12
60	7	9	11	12
55	7	9	10	11
50	6	8	10	11
45	6	7	9	10
40	5	7	9	10
35	4	6	8	9
30	4	5	7	9
25	2	4	6	9
20	2	4	6	8
15	1	3	5	8
10	1	2	3	6
5	0	0	1	5

Table 6.8. The MacArthur-Bates Communicative Development Inventory–III (CDI-III) fitted percentile values for Using Language—both sexes combined

%ile rank	Age (in months)			
	30–31	32–33	34–35	36–37
99	12	12	12	12
95	12	12	12	12
90	11	11	12	12
85	10	11	11	12
80	10	11	11	12
75	9	10	11	12
70	9	10	10	11
65	8	9	10	11
60	8	9	10	11
55	7	9	10	11
50	7	8	10	11
45	7	8	9	10
40	6	7	9	10
35	6	7	9	10
30	6	7	8	9
25	5	6	7	9
20	4	5	7	9
15	4	5	7	8
10	3	4	6	7
5	2	3	4	6

Table 6.9. The MacArthur-Bates Communicative Development Inventory–III (CDI-III) fitted percentile values for Using Language—girls

%ile rank	Age (in months)			
	30–31	32–33	34–35	36–37
99	12	12	12	12
95	12	12	12	12
90	11	12	12	12
85	11	11	11	12
80	11	11	11	12
75	10	11	11	12
70	10	11	11	12
65	9	10	10	11
60	9	9	10	11
55	9	9	10	11
50	8	9	10	11
45	7	9	10	11
40	7	8	9	10
35	7	8	9	10
30	6	8	9	10
25	6	7	8	9
20	6	7	8	9
15	5	6	8	9
10	4	5	7	8
5	3	4	5	7

Table 6.10. The MacArthur-Bates Communicative Development Inventory–III (CDI-III) fitted percentile values for Using Language—boys

%ile rank	Age (in months)			
	30–31	32–33	34–35	36–37
99	12	12	12	12
95	11	12	12	12
90	11	11	12	12
85	9	10	11	12
80	9	10	11	12
75	9	10	10	11
70	8	9	10	11
65	7	9	10	11
60	7	9	10	11
55	6	8	9	11
50	6	8	9	10
45	6	7	9	10
40	5	7	8	9
35	5	6	8	9
30	4	6	7	9
25	4	6	7	9
20	3	5	6	8
15	3	4	5	7
10	2	3	5	6
5	0	1	3	6

developing 36- to 37-month-olds. The correlation was .63 for PLS-3 Total Scale Score, .58 for the Auditory Comprehension score, and .47 for the Expressive Communication Score.

Mercure (1999) administered the Peabody Picture Vocabulary Test–Revised (PPVT-R; Dunn & Dunn, 1981) to 22 children between 36 and 39 months and then compared their scores with those on the CDI-III. PPVT-R scores were predicted at .50, .45, and .63 by CDI-III Vocabulary Checklist, Sentences, and Using Language, respectively.

Oliver and colleagues (2002) administered the McCarthy Scales of Children's Abilities (McCarthy, 1972) to 85 British children (50 boys and 35 girls, members of 43 twin pairs, 32–40 months of age), and their scores were compared with scores on a U.K. adaptation of the CDI-III Vocabulary Checklist measure. The correlation with the McCarthy Verbal Scale was .57 ($p < .001$). Interestingly, CDI-III Vocabulary Checklist was substantially correlated with all parts of the McCarthy, not just the verbal scale: .44 with Perceptual Performance, .52 with Quantitative, .52 with Memory, and .62 with the General Cognitive Index (GCI; all $p < .001$).

Finally, Feldman et al. (2005) compared CDI-III scores with the McCarthy Scales of Children's Abilities and PPVT-R scores for 113 children at age 3. All three components of the CDI-III form were moderately correlated with McCarthy Verbal Scale (.53, .56, and .52, respectively; all $p < .001$), the McCarthy

GCI (.53, .56, and .52; all $p < .001$), and the PPVT-R scores (.41, .49, and .49; all $p < .001$). Correlations with mean length of utterance from a 15-minute language sample were lower but still significant (.33, .42, and .31).

RESEARCH FINDINGS WITH THE CDI-III

As of 2006, several research studies using the CDI-III are underway. Two studies that have been completed and provide evidence for the usefulness of the measure are briefly described here. One concerns the balance of genetic and environmental influence on CDI-III measures; the other utilizes the CDI-III as a measure of the possible influence of otitis media on language development.

The Twins Early Development Study (TEDS; Plomin & Dale, 2000) is a very large, population-based study of early language and cognitive development. Dionne and colleagues (2003) examined Vocabulary Checklist and Sentences scores at ages 2 years (using the CDI: Words and Sentences form) and 3 years (using the CDI-III form) in a sample of 2,554 same-sex twins. Those born in 1994 (1,505 pairs) and in 1995 (1,049 pairs) were analyzed separately to serve as a replication. A comparison of the correlations of monozygotic and dizygotic twins demonstrated significant heritability for Vocabulary Checklist (.10 and .14 for the 1994 and 1995 cohorts, respectively) as well as substantially greater shared environmental influence (.84 and .82). The heritability for Sentences (.34, .29) was significantly higher than for Vocabulary Checklist, but it was still less than shared environmental influence (.47 and .56). There was a high genetic correlation (a measure of the overlap of genetic influences) between Vocabulary Checklist and Sentences at age 3 in both cohorts (.89 and .63). Finally, longitudinal analyses provided evidence for both lexical and syntactic bootstrapping.

Feldman and colleagues (2003) used the CDI-III along with other measures to evaluate the outcome for children with a history of ear infections, specifically otitis media with middle-ear effusion (MEE), within a sample of 621 children. The study utilized a prospective design and included careful monitoring of ear infections. At ages 1, 2, and 3 years, parents completed the CDI: Words and Gestures form, CDI: Words and Sentences form, and CDI-III form, respectively. At age 1, only the mean number of gestures produced on the CDI: Words and Gestures form was related ($r = -.101$) to cumulative days with MEE. At age 2, there was a weak relation with the CDI: Words and Sentences form: $r = -.117$, $-.162$, and $-.119$ for Expressive Vocabulary, Examples/mean length of three longest sentences (M3L), and Complexity, respectively. At age 3, the CDI-III measures were significantly and moderately related to cumulative days with MEE: $-.187$, $-.229$, and $-.248$ for Vocabulary Checklist, Sentences, and Using Language, respectively.

Both behavioral genetic research and research on early environmental influence, such as ear infections, typically require large samples in order to differentiate the sources of influence. Parent report measures such as the CDI-III are especially useful in studies of these types.

CONCLUSIONS

The CDI-III form is still at a relatively early stage of development, when compared with the CDI: Words and Gestures and CDI: Words and Sentences forms, which have a more extensive history of norming and revision. The validity evidence for the CDI-III, although not yet conclusive, is sufficiently encouraging to justify making the instrument available for wider use. As with the earlier versions of the other CDIs, use by the research and clinical communities will yield more complete information about the appropriate uses and limitations of the instrument.

REFERENCES

Acredolo, L.P., & Goodwyn, S.W. (1985). Symbolic gesturing in language development: A case study. *Human Development, 28,* 40–49.

Acredolo, L.P., & Goodwyn, S.W. (1988). Symbolic gesturing in normal infants. *Child Development, 59,* 450–456.

Anastasi, A. (1988). *Psychological testing* (6th ed.). New York: Macmillan.

Anderson, R. (1995). Spanish morphological and syntactic development. In H. Kayser (Ed.), *Bilingual speech-language pathology: A Hispanic focus* (pp. 41–72). San Diego: Singular Publishing Group.

Arriaga, R.I., Fenson, L., Cronan, T., & Pethick, S. (1998). Scores on the MacArthur Communicative Development Inventory of children from low- and middle-income families. *Applied Psycholinguistics, 19*(2), 209–223.

Bangs, T.E., & Dodson, S. (1979). *Birth to Three Developmental Scale.* Boston: Teaching Resources Corporation.

Bates, E., Benigni, L., Bretherton, I., Camaioni, L., & Volterra, V. (1979). *The emergence of symbols: Cognition and communication in infancy.* San Diego: Academic Press.

Bates, E., Bretherton, I., & Snyder, L. (1988). *From first words to grammar: Individual differences and dissociable mechanisms.* New York: Cambridge University Press.

Bates, E., Camaioni, L., & Volterra, V. (1975). The acquisition of performatives prior to speech. *Merrill-Palmer Quarterly, 21*(3), 205–226.

Bates, E., Dale, P.S., & Thal, D. (1995). Individual differences and their implications for theories of language development. In P. Fletcher & B. MacWhinney (Eds.), *Handbook of child language* (pp. 96–151). Oxford, United Kingdom: Blackwell.

Bates, E., & Goodman, J.C. (1999). On the emergence of grammar from the lexicon. B. MacWhinney (Ed.), *The emergence of language* (pp. 29–70). Mahwah, NJ: Lawrence Erlbaum Associates.

Bates, E., Marchman, V., Thal, D., Fenson, L., Dale, P., & Reznick, J.S., et al. (1994). Developmental and stylistic variation in the composition of early vocabulary. *Journal of Child Language, 21*(1), 85–123.

Bates, E., Thal, D., Whitesell, K., Fenson, L., & Oakes, L. (1989). Integrating language and gesture in infancy. *Developmental Psychology, 25*(6), 1004–1019.

Bauer, D., Goldfield, B., & Reznick, J. (2002). Alternative approaches to analyzing individual differences in the rate of early vocabulary development. *Applied Psycholinguistics, 23,* 313–315.

Bayley, N. (1993). *Bayley Scales of Infant Development–Second Edition.* San Antonio, TX: Harcourt Assessment.

Beeghly, M., Jernberg, E., & Burrows, E. (1989, April), *Validity of the Early Language Inventory (ELI) for use with 25-month-olds.* Paper presented at the Society for Research in Child Development annual meeting, Kansas City, MO.

Benedict, H. (1979). Early lexical development: Comprehension and production. *Journal of Child Language, 6*(2), 183–200.

Berko, J. (1958). The child's learning of English morphology. *Word, 14*, 150–177.

Bishop, D.V.M. (1997). *Uncommon understanding: Development and disorders of language comprehension in children.* East Sussex, United Kingdom: Psychology Press.

Bloom, L., & Lahey, M. (1978). *Language development and language disorders.* New York: John Wiley & Sons.

Bornstein, M.H., & Cote, L.R. (2004). Mothers' parenting cognitions in cultures of origin, acculturating cultures, and cultures of destination. *Child Development, 75*(1), 221–235.

Bornstein, M.H., & Haynes, O.M. (1998). Vocabulary competence in early childhood: Measurement, latent construct, and predictive validity. *Child Development, 69*(3), 654–671.

Bornstein, M.H., Haynes, O.M., & Painter, K. (1998). Sources of child vocabulary competence: A multivariate model. *Journal of Child Language, 25*(2), 367–393.

Bornstein, M.H., Tamis LeMonda, C.S., & Haynes, O.M. (1999). First words in the second year: Continuity, stability, and models of concurrent and predictive correspondence in vocabulary and verbal responsiveness across age and context. *Infant Behavior and Development, 22*(1), 65–85.

Braine, M.D.S. (1976). Children's first word combinations. *Monographs of the Society for Research in Child Development, 41*(Serial No. 164).

Bretherton, I. (1984). Representing the social world in symbolic play: Reality and fantasy. In I. Bretherton (Ed.), *Symbolic play: The development of social understanding* (pp. 3–41). San Diego: Academic Press.

Bretherton, I., & Bates, E. (1984). The development of representation from 10 to 28 months: Differential stability of language and symbolic play. In R. Emde & R. Harmon (Eds.), *Continuities and discontinuities in development* (pp. 229–259). New York: Kluwer Academic/Plenum Publishers.

Brigance, A.H. (1991). *Brigance Inventory of Early Development–Revised.* North Billerica, MA: Curriculum Associates.

Brown, R. (1973). *A first language.* Cambridge, MA: Harvard University Press.

Bruner, J. (1977). Early social interactions and language acquisition. In H. Schaffer (Ed.), *Studies in mother–infant interaction* (pp. 271–289). San Diego: Academic Press.

Butterworth, G., & Morissette, P. (1996). Onset of pointing and the acquisition of language in infancy. *Journal of Reproductive and Infant Psychology, 14*(3), 219–231.

Burchinal, M., & Applebaum, M.I. (1991). Estimating individual developmental functions: Methods and their assumptions. *Child Development, 62*, 23–41.

Bybee, J., & Slobin, D. (1982). Rules and schemas in the development and use of the English past tense. *Language, 58*, 211–226.

Bzoch, K.R., & League, R. (1991). *Receptive-Expressive Emergent Language Test, Second Edition.* Austin, TX: PRO-ED.

Capirci, O., Iverson, J., Pizzutto, E., & Volterra, V. (1996). Gestures and words during the transition to two-word speech. *Journal of Child Language, 23*(3), 645–673.

Carpenter, M., Nagell, K., & Tomasello, M. (1998). Social cognition, joint attention, and communicative competence from 9–15 months. *Monographs of the Society for Research in Child Development, 63* (Serial No. 255).

Carrillo Aranguren, G., Jackson-Maldonado, D., Thal, D., & Flores, M. (1997, June). *Language in lower income Spanish-speaking toddlers: Can standard assessment measures be used?* Poster session presented at the symposium on Research in Child Language Disorders, Madison, WI.

Carson, C.P., Klee, T., Carson, D., & Hime, L. (2003). Phonological profiles of 2-year-olds with delayed language development: Predicting clinical outcomes at age 3. *American Journal of Speech-Language Pathology, 12*, 28–39.

Caselli, M.C. (1990). Communicative gestures and first words. In V. Volterra & C.J. Erting (Eds.), *From gesture to language in hearing and deaf children* (pp. 56–67). New York: Springer-Verlag.

Caselli, M.C., & Casadio, P. (1995). *Il Primo vocabulario del bambino* [Children's early vocabulary]. Milan, Italy: France Angeli.

Caselli, M.C., Vicari, S., Longobardi, E., Lami, L., Pizzoli, C., & Stella, G. (1998). Gestures and words in early development of children with Down syndrome. *Journal of Speech, Language, and Hearing Research, 41*, 1125–1135.

Charman, T., Drew, A., Baird, C., & Baird, G. (2003). Measuring early language development in preschool children with autism spectrum disorder using the MacArthur Communicative Development Inventory (Infant Form). *Journal of Child Language, 30*, 213–236.

Crais, E.R. (1995). Expanding the repertoire of tools and techniques for assessing the communication skills of infants and toddlers. *American Journal of Speech-Language Pathology, 4*(3), 47–59.

Dale, P.S. (1990). *Parent report and the growth of MLU*. Unpublished manuscript.

Dale, P.S. (1991). The validity of a parent report measure of vocabulary and syntax at 24 months. *Journal of Speech and Hearing Sciences, 34*(3), 565–571.

Dale, P.S. (1996). Parent report assessment of language and communication. In S.F. Warren & J. Reichle (Series Eds.) & K.N. Cole, P.S. Dale, & D.J. Thal (Vol. Eds.), *Communication and language intervention series: Vol. 6. Advances in assessment of communication and language* (pp. 161–182). Baltimore: Paul H. Brookes Publishing Co.

Dale, P.S., Bates, E., Reznick, S., & Morisset, C. (1989). The validity of a parent report instrument of child language at 20 months. *Journal of Child Language, 16*(2), 239–250.

Dale, P.S., Dionne, G., Eley, T., & Plomin, R. (2000). Lexical and grammatical development: A behavioral genetic perspective. *Journal of Child Language, 27*, 619–642.

Dale, P.S., & Fenson, L. (1996). Lexical development norms for young children. *Behavior Research Methods, Instruments, & Computers, 28*, 125–127.

Dale, P.S., Fenson, L., & Thal, D. (1993). *Some suggestions for the adaptation of the MacArthur Communicative Development Inventories to additional languages*. Unpublished manuscript.

Delgado-Gaitan, C., & Trueba, T. (1991). *Crossing cultural borders*. New York: Falmer Press.

Demuth, K. (1992). The acquisition of Sesotho. In D.I. Slobin (Ed.), *The cross-linguistic study of language acquisition* (Vol. 3, pp. 557–638). Mahwah, NJ: Lawrence Erlbaum Associates.

deVilliers, J.G., & deVilliers, P.A. (1973). Development of the use of word order in comprehension. *Journal of Psycholinguistic Research, 2*, 331–341.

Dionne, G., Dale, P.S., Boivin, M., & Plomin, R. (2003). Genetic evidence for bidirectional effects of early lexical and grammatical development. *Child Development, 74*, 394–412.

Dollaghan, C.A., Campbell, T.F., Paradise, J.L., Feldman, H.M., Jansoky, J.E., Pitcairn, D.N., et al. (1999). Maternal education and measures of early speech and language. *Journal of Speech, Language, and Hearing Research, 42*(6), 1432–1443.

Dromi, E. (1987). *Early lexical development*. New York: Cambridge University Press.

Dunn, L.M., & Dunn, L.M. (1981). *Peabody Picture Vocabulary Test–Revised*. Circle Pines, MN: AGS Publishing.

Dunn, L.M., & Dunn, L.M. (1997). *Peabody Picture Vocabulary Test–Third Edition*. Circle Pines, MN: AGS Publishing.

Education of the Handicapped Act Amendments of 1986, PL 99-457, 20 U.S.C. §§ 1400 *et seq.*

Edwards, S., Fletcher, P., Garman, M., Hughes, A., Letts, C., & Sinka, I. (1997). *Reynell Developmental Language Scales (RDLS)–Third Edition*. London: NFER-Nelson.

Farver, J.M. (1993). Cultural differences in scaffolding pretend play. In K. MacDonald (Ed.), *Parent–child play: Descriptions and implications* (pp. 349–366). Albany, NY: SUNY Press.

Feldman, H.M., Dale, P.S., Campbell, T.F., Colborn, D.K., Kurs-Lasky, M., & Rockette, H.E., et al. (2005). Concurrent and predictive validity of parent reports of child language at ages 2 and 3 years. *Child Development, 76*, 856–868.

Feldman, H.M., Dollaghan, C.A., Campbell, T.F., Colborn, D.K., Janosky, J., Kurs-Lasky, M., et al. (2003). Parent-reported language skills in relation to otitis media during the first three years of life. *Journal of Speech-Language-Hearing Research, 46*, 273–287.

Feldman, H.M., Dollaghan, C.A., Campbell, T.F., Kurs-Lasky, M., Janosky, J.E., & Paradise, J.L. (2000). Measurement properties of the MacArthur Communicative Development Inventories at ages one and two years. *Child Development, 71*(2), 310–322.

Fenson, L., Bates, E., Dale, P., Goodman, J., Reznick, J.S., & Thal, D. (2000). Measuring variability in early child language: Don't shoot the messenger. *Child Development, 71*(2), 323–328.

Fenson, L. Dale, P.S., Reznick, J.S., Bates, E., Thal, D.J., & Pethick, S.J. (1994). Variability in early communicative development. *Monographs of the Society for Research in Child Development, 59*(5, Serial No. 242).

Fenson, L. Dale, P.S., Reznick, J.S., Thal, D., Bates, E., Hartung, J.P., et al. (1993). *MacArthur Communicative Development Inventories: Users guide and technical manual.* Baltimore: Paul H. Brookes Publishing Co. (Original copyright assigned 1992)

Fenson, L., Kagan, J., Kearsley, R.B., & Zelazo, P.R. (1976). The developmental progression of manipulative play in the first two years. *Child Development, 47*(1), 232–236.

Fenson, L., Pethick, S., Renda, C., Cox, J.L., Dale, P.S., & Reznick, J.S. (2000). Short-form versions of the MacArthur Communicative Development Inventories. *Applied Psycholinguistics, 21*(1), 95–116.

Fenson, L., & Ramsey, D.S. (1980). Decentration and integration of play in the second year of life. *Child Development, 52,* 171–178.

Fenson, L., Thal, D., & Bates, E. (1990). *Normed values for the "Early Language Inventory" and three associated parent report forms for language assessment* (Tech. Rep.). San Diego: San Diego State University.

Fischel, J., Whitehurst, G., Caufield, M., & Debaryshe, B. (1989). Language growth in children with expressive language delay. *Pediatrics, 82,* 218–227.

Frankenburg, W.K., Dodds, J.B., Fandal, A.W., Kazuk, E., & Cohrs, M. (1975). *Denver Developmental Screening Test* (Rev. ed.), Denver, CO: Denver Developmental Materials.

Garcia Coll, C.T. (1990). Developmental outcomes of minority infants: A process-oriented look into our beginnings. *Child Development, 61,* 270–289.

Gardner, M.F. (1981). *Expressive One-Word Picture Vocabulary Test (EOWPVT).* Novato, CA: Academic Therapy Publications.

Gershkoff-Stowe, L., & Smith, L.B (1997). A curvilinear trend in naming errors as a function of early vocabulary growth. *Cognitive Psychology, 34*(1), 37–71.

Gersten, M., Coster, W., Schneider-Rosen, K., Carlson, V., & Cicchetti, D. (1986). The socio-emotional bases of communicative functioning: Quality of attachment, language development, and early maltreatment. In M.E. Lamb, A.L. Brown, & B. Rogoff (Eds.), *Advances in developmental psychology* (Vol. 4, pp. 105–151). Mahwah, NJ: Erlbaum Associates.

Girolametto, L., Pearce, P.S., & Weitzman, E. (1996). Interactive focus stimulation for toddlers with expressive vocabulary delays. *Journal of Speech and Hearing Research, 39*(6), 1274–1283.

Girolametto, L., Pearce, P.S., & Weitzman, E. (1997). Effects of lexical intervention on the phonology of late talkers. *Journal of Speech, Language, and Hearing Research, 40*(2), 338–348.

Girolametto, L., Weitzman, E., Wiigs, M., & Pearce, P.S. (1999). The relationship between maternal language measures and language development in toddlers with expressive vocabulary delays. *American Journal of Speech-Language Pathology, 8*(4), 364–374.

Gleitman, L.R., & Gleitman, H. (1970). *Phrase and paraphrase.* New York: W.W. Norton.

Goldin-Meadow, S., & Morford, M. (1985). Gesture in early child language: Studies of deaf and hearing children. *Merrill-Palmer Quarterly, 31*(2), 145–176.

Gutierrez-Clellen, V.F. (1996). Language diversity: Implications for assessment. In S.F. Warren & J. Reichle (Series Eds.) & K.N. Cole, P.S. Dale, & D.J. Thal (Vol. Eds.), *Communication and language intervention series: Vol. 6. Advances in assessment of communication and language* (pp. 29–56). Baltimore: Paul H. Brookes Publishing Co.

Gutierrez-Clellen, V.F., Restrepo, M.A., Bedore, L., Peña, E., & Anderson, R. (2000). Language sample analysis in Spanish-speaking children: Methodological considerations. *Language, Speech, and Hearing Services in Schools, 31,* 88–89.

Hart, B., & Risley, T.R. (1995). *Meaningful differences in the everyday experience of young American children.* Baltimore: Paul H. Brookes Publishing Co.

Heath, S.B. (1983). *Ways with words: Language, life and work in communities and classrooms.* New York: Cambridge University.

Hedrick, D.L., Prather, E.M., & Tobin, A.R. (1984). *Sequenced Inventory of Communication Development–Revised Edition (SICD-R).* Seattle: University of Washington Press.

Heilmann, J., Weismer, S.E,. Evans, J., & Hollar, C. (2005). Utility of the MacArthur-Bates communicative development inventory in identifying language abilities of late-talking and typically developing toddlers. *American Journal of Speech-Language Pathology, 14*(1), 40–51.

Hernández-Pina, F. (1984). *Teorias psico-sociolinguisticas y su aplicacion a la adquisicion del espanol como lengua materna* [Psycholinguistic theories and their application to Spanish as a first language]. Madrid, Spain: Siglo XXI Editores.

Horwitz, S.H., Irwin, J.R., Briggs-Gowan, M.J., Heenan, J.M.B., Mendoza, J., & Carter, A.S. (2003). Language delay in a community cohort of young children. *Journal of the American Academy of Child and Adolescent Psychiatry, 42,* 932–940.

Huebner, C.E. (2000). Community-based support for preschool readiness among children in poverty. *Journal of Education for Students Placed at Risk, 5*(3), 291–314.

Individuals with Disabilities Education Act (IDEA) Amendments of 1997, PL 105-17, 20 U.S.C. §§ 1400 *et seq.*

Individuals with Disabilities Education Improvement Act of 2004, PL 108-446, 20 U.S.C. §§ 1400 *et seq.*

Irwin, J.R., Carter, A.S., & Briggs-Gowan, M.J. (2002). The social-emotional development of 'late-talking' toddlers. *Journal of the American Academy of Child and Adolescent Psychiatry, 41,* 1324–1332.

Iverson, J., Capirci, O., & Caselli, M.C. (1994). From communication to language in two modalities. *Cognitive Development, 9*(1), 23–43.

Jackson, S.C. (1996). *Family and professional congruence in communication assessment of preschool boys with Fragile X syndrome (mental retardation).* Unpublished doctoral dissertation, University of North Carolina at Chapel Hill.

Jackson-Maldonado, D. (1994). *Lenguaje y Cognacion en los primeros Anos de Vida: Fase 2* [Language and cognition in the first years of life: Phase 2]. Project financed by the Consejo Nacional de Ciencia y Tecnologia (CONACYT), Mexico City, Mexico.

Jackson-Maldonado, D. (1997). *Early communicative abilities of Spanish-speaking children: Vocabulary, phrases and gestures.* Seminar presented at the Research Symposium on Language Diversity in Multicultural Communication Sciences and Disorders, Austin, TX.

Jackson-Maldonado, D., Thal, D.J., Fenson, L., Marchman, V.A., Newton, T., & Conboy, B. (2003). *MacArthur Inventarios del Desarrollo de Habilidades Comunicatives Users Guide and Technical Manual.* Baltimore: Paul H. Brookes Publishing Co.

Jackson-Maldonado, D., Thal, D., Marchman, V., Bates, E., & Gutierrez-Clellen, V. (1993). Early lexical development of Spanish-speaking infants and toddlers. *Journal of Child Language, 20*(3), 523–549.

Kayser, H. (1995). Intervention with children from linguistically and culturally diverse backgrounds. In S.F. Warren & J. Reichle (Series Eds.) & M.E. Fey, J. Windsor, & S.W. Warren (Vol. Eds.), *Communication and language intervention series: Vol. 5. Language intervention: Preschool through the elementary years* (pp. 315–331). Baltimore: Paul H. Brookes Publishing Co.

Klee, T., Carson, D., Gavin, W., Hall, L., Kent, A., & Reece, S. (1998). Concurrent and predictive validity of an early language screening program. *Journal of Speech, Language, and Hearing Research, 41,* 627–641.

Klee, T., Pearce, K., & Carson, D. (2000). Improving the positive predictive value of screening for developmental language disorder. *Journal of Speech, Language, and Hearing Disorders, 43,* 821–833.

Laasko, M.-L., Poikkeus, A.-M., Eklund, K., & Lyytinen, P. (1999). Social interactional behaviors and symbolic play competence as predictors of language development and their associations with maternal attention-directing strategies. *Infant Behavior and Development, 22*(4), 541–556.

Lahey, M. (1988). *Language disorders and language development.* New York: Macmillan.

Langdon, H.W. (1992a). Language communication and sociocultural patterns in Hispanic families. In H.W. Langdon & L.L. Cheng (Eds.), *Hispanic children and adults with communication disorders: Assessment and intervention* (pp. 99–131). Gaithersburg, MD: Aspen Publishers.

Langdon, H.W. (1992b). Speech and language assessment of LEP/bilingual Hispanic students. In H.W. Langdon & L.L. Cheng (Eds.), *Hispanic children and adults with communication disorders: Assessment and Intervention* (pp. 201–271). Gaithersburg, MD: Aspen Publishers.

Laosa, L. (1982). School, occupation, culture, and family: The impact of parental schooling on the parent-child relationship. *Journal of Educational Psychology, 74*(6), 791–827.

Laosa, L.M. (1984). *Ethnic, socioeconomic, and home language influences upon early performance on measures of abilities.* Princeton, NJ: Educational Testing Service.

Lawrence, C.W. (1992). Assessing the use of age-equivalent scores in clinical management. *Language Speech and Hearing Services in Schools, 23*(1), 6–8.

Leonard, L.B. (1998). *Children with specific language impairment.* Cambridge, MA: The MIT Press.

Leopold, W.F. (1949). *Speech development of a bilingual child: A linguist's record* (Vol. 3). Evanston, IL: Northwestern University Press.

Llorach, E.A. (1976). La adquisición del lenguaje por el niño. In A. Martinez (Ed.), *Tratado de lenguaje* (pp. 9–42). Buenos Aires, Argentina: Nueva Visión.

Locke, A. (1978). *Action, gesture, and symbol.* San Diego: Academic Press.

López Ornat, S., Fernandez, A., Gallo, P., & Mariscal, S. (1994). *La adquisicion de la lengua Espanola* [Acquisition of the Spanish language]. Madrid, Spain: Siglo XXI Editores.

Lund, N.J., & Duchan, J.F. (1988). *Assessing children's language in naturalistic contexts* (2nd ed.). Upper Saddle River, NJ: Prentice-Hall.

Lyman, H. (1998). *Test scores and what they mean* (6th ed.). Boston: Allyn & Bacon.

Lyytinen, P., Poikkeus, A.M., Leiwo, M., Ahonen, T., & Lyytinen, H. (1996). Parents as informants of their child's vocal and early language development. *Early Child Development and Care, 126,* 15–25.

Magill-Evans, J., & Harrison, M.J. (1999). Parent–child interactions and development of toddlers born preterm. *Western Journal of Nursing Research, 21*(3), 292–307.

Marchman, C., & Bates, E. (1994). Continuity in lexical and morphological development: A test of the critical mass hypothesis. *Journal of Child Language, 21,* 331–366.

Marchman, V.A., & Martínez-Sussmann, C. (2002). Concurrent validity of caregiver/parent report measures of language for children who are learning both English and Spanish. *Journal of Speech, Language, and Hearing Research, 45*(5), 993–997.

Marchman, V.A., Martínez-Sussmann, C., & Dale, P.S. (2004). The language-specific nature of grammatical development: Evidence from bilingual language learners. *Developmental Science, 7*(2), 212–224.

Marcus, G.F., Pinker, S., Ullman, M., Hollander, M., Rosen, T.J., & Xu, F. (1992). Overregularization in language acquisition. *Monographs of the Society for Research in Child Development, 57*(4, Serial No. 228).

Mattes, L.J., & Omark, D.R. (1991). *Speech and language assessment for the bilingual handicapped* (2nd ed.). Oceanside, CA: Academic Communication Associates.

Mayne, A.M., Yoshinaga-Itano, C., Sedey, A.L., & Carey, A. (2000a). Expressive vocabulary development of infants and toddlers who are deaf or hard of hearing. *The Volta Review, 100*(5), 1–28.

Mayne, A.M., Yoshinaga-Itano, C., Sedey, A.L., & Carey, A. (2000b). Receptive vocabulary development of infants and toddlers who are deaf or hard of hearing. *The Volta Review, 100*(5), 29–52.

McCall, R., Eichorn, D., & Hogarty, P. (1977). Transitions in early mental development. *Monographs of the Society for Research in Child Development, 42*(3, Serial No. 171).

McCune-Nicolich, L., & Fenson, L. (1984). Methodological issues in studying early pretend play. In T.D. Yawkey & A.D. Pellegrini (Eds.), *Child's play: Developmental and applied.* Mahwah, NJ: Lawrence Erlbaum Associates.

McCarthy, D.A. (1972). *Manual for the McCarthy Scales of Children's Abilities.* San Antonio, TX: Harcourt Assessment.

McGrath, P.J., Rosmus, C., Canfield, C., Campbell, M.A., & Hennigar, A. (1998). Behaviours caregivers use to determine pain in non-verbal, cognitively impaired individuals. *Developmental Medicine and Child Neurology, 40*(5), 340–343.

Mercure, A.M. (1999). *The quality of parent–child bookreading interaction: Parental attitudes and child engagement.* Unpublished honors thesis, University of Washington, Seattle.

Mervis, C.B., & Robinson, B.F. (2000). Expressive vocabulary ability of toddlers with Williams syndrome or Down syndrome: A comparison. *Developmental Neuropsychology, 17*(1), 111–126.

Miller, J.F. (1981). *Assessing language production in children: Experimental procedures.* Baltimore: University Park Press.

Miller, J.F., Sedey, A.L., & Miolo, G. (1995). Validity of parent report measures of vocabulary development for children with Down syndrome. *Journal of Speech and Hearing Research, 38,* 1037–1044.

Nelson, K. (1973). Structure and strategy in learning to talk. *Monographs of the Society for Research in Child Development, 48*(Serial No. 149).

Nott, P., Cowan, R., Brown, M.P., & Wigglesworth, G. (2003). Assessment of language skills in young children with profound hearing loss under two years of age. *Journal of Deaf Studies and Deaf Education, 8*(4), 401–421.

O'Hanlon, L., & Thal, D. (1991, November). *MacArthur CDI/Toddlers: Validation for language impaired children.* Paper presented at the American Speech-Language Hearing Association annual convention, Atlanta, GA.

Oliver, B., Dale, P.S., Saudino, K.J., Petrill, S.A., Pike, A., & Plomin, R. (2002). The validity of a parent-based assessment of cognitive abilities in three-year-olds. *Early Child Development & Care, 17,* 337–348.

Paul, R. (1996). Clinical implications of the natural history of slow expressive language development. *American Journal of Speech-Language Pathology, 5*(2), 5–21.

Paul, R. (1997). Understanding language delay: A reply to van Kleeck, Gillam, and Davis. *American Journal of Speech-Language Pathology, 6*(2), 40–49.

Pearson, B.Z., Fernandez, S.C., & Oller, D.K. (1993). Lexical development in bilingual infants and toddlers: Comparison to monolingual norms. *Language Learning, 43*(1), 93–120.

Pearson, B.Z., Fernandez, S., & Oller, D.K. (1993/1995). Lexical development in bilingual infants and toddlers: Comparison to monolingual norms. In B. Harley (Ed.), *Lexical issues in language learning* (pp. 31–57). Toronto: Ontario Institute for Studies in Education. (Reprinted from *Language Learning, 43*[1], 93–120.)

Pearson, B.Z., Fernandez, S., & Oller, D.K. (1995). Cross-language synonyms in the lexicons of bilingual infants: One language or two? *Journal of Child Language, 22,* 345–368.

Perez, M., & Castro, J. (1988). Fenomenos transicionales en el acceso al lenguaje. *Infancia y aprendizaje, 43,* 13–36.

Piaget, J. (1952). *The origins of intelligence in children.* New York: International Universities Press.

Piaget, J. (1962). *Play, dreams, and imitation in childhood.* New York: W.W. Norton.

Plomin, R., & Dale, P.S. (2000). Genetics and early language development: A UK study of twins. In D.V.M. Bishop & L.B. Leonard (Eds.), *Speech and language impairments in children: Causes, characteristics, intervention, and outcome* (pp. 35–51). Philadelphia: Taylor & Francis.

Plomin, R., Price, T.S., Eley, T.C., Dale, P.S., & Stevenson, J. (2002). Associations between behavior problems and verbal and nonverbal cognitive abilities and disabilities in early childhood. *Journal of Child Psychology and Psychiatry, 43,* 619–633.

Price, T.S., Eley, T.C., Dale, P.S., Stevenson, J., & Plomin, R. (2000). Genetic and environmental covariation between verbal and non-verbal cognitive development in infancy. *Child Development, 71,* 948–959.

Rescorla, L. (1989). The Language Development Survey: A screening tool for delayed language in toddlers. *Journal of Speech and Hearing Disorders, 54*(4), 587–599.

Rescorla, L. (1991). Identifying expressive language delay at age two. *Topics in Language Disorders, 11*(4), 14–20.

Rescorla, L. (2000). Do late-talking toddlers turn out to have reading difficulties a decade later? *Annals of Dyslexia, 50,* 87–102.

Rescorla, L., & Alley, A. (2001). Validation of the Language Development Survey (LDS): A parent report tool for identifying language delay in toddlers. *Journal of Speech, Language, and Hearing Research, 44*(2), 434–445.

Rescorla, L., & Schwartz, E. (1990). Outcome of toddlers with specific expressive language delay. *Applied Psycholinguistics, 11*(4), 393–407.

Reznick, J.S. (1982). *The development of perceptual and lexical categories in the human infant.* Unpublished doctoral dissertation, University of Colorado, Boulder.

Reznick, J.S. (1990). Visual preference as a test of infant word comprehension. *Applied Psycholinguistics, 11,* 145–166.

Reznick, J.S., & Schwartz, B.B. (2001). When is an assessment an intervention? Parent perception of infant intentionality and language. *Journal of the American Academy of Child and Adolescent Psychiatry, 40,* 11–17.

Reynell, J., & Gruber, C. (1990). *Reynell Developmental Language Scales: U.S. Edition.* Los Angeles: Western Psychological Services.

Reynell, J., & Huntley, M. (1985). *Reynell Developmental Language Scales (RDLS)–Second Version: British Edition.* London: NFER-Nelson.

Roberts, J.E., Burchinal, M., & Durham, M. (1999). Parents' report of vocabulary and grammatical development of African American preschoolers: Child and environmental associations. *Child Development, 70*(1), 92–106.

Robertson, S.B., & Weismer, S.E. (1999). Effects of treatment on linguistic and social skills in toddlers with delayed language development. *Journal of Speech, Language, and Hearing Research, 42*(5), 1234–1248.

Rodrigue, S.R. (2001). *Assessment of language comprehension and production in children from low-income and middle-income homes: Parent report versus child performance.* Unpublished master's thesis, San Diego State University.

Rollins, P.R. (2003). Caregivers' contingent comments to 9-month-old infants: Relationships with later language. *Applied Psycholinguistics, 24*(2) 221–234.

Rollins, P.R., & Snow, C.E. (1998). Shared attention and grammatical development in typical children and children with autism. *Journal of Child Language, 25*(3), 653–673.

Roopnarine, J., Johnson, J., & Hooper, F. (Eds.). (1994). *Children's play in diverse cultures.* Albany, NY: SUNY Press.

Rossetti, L. (1995). *The Rossetti Infant-Toddler Language Scale: A measure of communication and interaction.* East Moline, IL: LinguiSystems.

Sattler, J.M. (1988). *Assessment of children* (3rd edition). San Diego: Author.

Saxon, T.F. (1997). A longitudinal study of mother–infant interaction and later language competence. *First Language, 17,* 271–281.

Scarborough, H. (1990). Index of Productive Syntax. *Applied Psycholinguistics, 11,* 1–22.

Scherer, N.J. (1999). The speech and language status of toddlers with cleft lip and/or palate following early vocabulary intervention. *American Journal of Speech-Language Pathology, 8*(1), 81–93.

Simcock, G., & Hayne, H. (2003). Age-related changes in verbal and nonverbal memory during early childhood. *Developmental Psychology, 5,* 805–814.

Snyder, L. (1975). *Pragmatics in language-deficient children: Prelinguistic and early verbal performatives and presuppositions.* Unpublished doctoral dissertation, University of Colorado, Boulder.

Snyder, L., Bates, E., & Bretherton, I. (1981). Content and context in early language development. *Journal of Child Language, 8*(3), 565–582.

Snyder, L.E., & Scherer, N. (2004). The development of symbolic play and language in toddlers with cleft palate. *American Journal of Speech-Language Pathology, 13,* 66–80.

Stallings, L.M., Gao, S., & Svirsky, M.A. (2002). Assessing the language abilities of pediatric cochlear implant users across a broad range of ages and performance abilities. *The Volta Review, 102*(4), 215–235.

Stern, C., & Stern, W. (1907). *Die kindersprache: Eine psychologische und sprachtheoretische Untersuchung.* Leipzig, Germany: Berth.

Stone, W.L., & Yoder, P.J. (2001). Predicting spoken language level in children with autism spectrum disorders. *Autism, 5,* 341–361.

Tamis-LeMonda, C., & Bornstein, M. (1989). Habituation and maternal encouragement of attention in infancy as predictors of toddler language, play, and representational competence. *Child Development, 60,* 738–751.

Tamis-LeMonda, C., & Bornstein, M. (1990). Language, play, and attention at one year. *Infant Behavior and Development, 13*(1), 85–98.

Terrell, B., & Schwartz, R. (1988). Object transformations in the play of language-impaired children. *Journal of Speech and Hearing Disorders, 53*(4), 459–456.

Terrell, B., Schwartz, R., Prelock, P., & Messick, C. (1984). Symbolic play in normal and language impaired children. *Journal of Speech and Hearing Research, 27*(3), 424–429.

Thal, D. (2000). *Late-talking toddlers: Are they at risk?* San Diego: San Diego State University Press.

Thal, D., & Bates, E. (1988). Language and gesture in late talkers. *Journal of Speech and Hearing Research, 31*(1), 115–123.

Thal, D., & Bates, E. (1989). Language development in early childhood. *Pediatric Annals, 18,* 299–306.

Thal, D.J., Bates, E., Zappia, M.J., & Oroz, M. (1996). Ties between lexical and grammatical development: Evidence from early talkers. *Journal of Child Language, 23*(2), 349–368.

Thal, D., DesJardin, J. & Eisenberg, L. (2006). *Validity of the MacArthur-Bates Communicative Development Inventory for measuring language abilities in children with cochlear implants.* Manuscript under review.

Thal, D., & Dughi. (1990). Unpublished honors thesis, University of California, San Diego.

Thal, D., & Hoffman. (1990). Unpublished honors thesis, University of California, San Diego.

Thal, D., Jackson-Maldonado, D., & Acosta, D. (2000). Validity of a parent report measure of vocabulary and grammar for Spanish-speaking toddlers. *Journal of Speech, Language, and Hearing Research, 43,* 1087–1100.

Thal, D., Jackson-Maldonado, D., & Fenson, L. (1999, July). *Fundacion MacArthur: Inventario del Desarollo de Habilidades Communicativas: Norms and validation studies.* Poster session presented at the eighth International Conference for the Study of Child Language, San Sebastian, Spain.

Thal, D.J., & Katich, J. (1996). Predicaments in early identification of specific language impairment: Does the early bird always catch the worm? In S.F. Warren & J. Reichle (Series Eds.) & K.N. Cole, P.S. Dale, & D.J. Thal (Vol. Eds.), *Communication and language intervention series: Vol. 6. Advances in assessment of communication and language* (pp. 1–28). Baltimore: Paul H. Brookes Publishing Co.

Thal, D.J., O'Hanlon, L., Clemmons, M., & Fralin, L. (1999). Validity of a parent report measure of vocabulary and syntax for preschool children with language impairment. *Journal of Speech, Language, and Hearing Research, 42,* 482–496.

Thal, D.J., Reilly, J., Seibert, L., Jeffries, R., & Fenson, J. (2004). Language development in children at risk for language impairment: cross-population comparisons. *Brain and Language, 88*(2), 167–179

Thal, D.J., & Tobias, S. (1992). Communicative gestures in children with delayed onset of oral expressive vocabulary. *Journal of Speech and Hearing Research, 35*(6) 1281–1289.

Thal, D.J., & Tobias, S. (1994). Relationships between language and gesture in normal developing and late-talking toddlers. *Journal of Speech and Hearing Research, 37*(1), 157–170.

Thal, D.J., Tobias, S., & Morrison, D. (1991). Language and gesture in late talkers: A one year follow-up. *Journal of Speech and Hearing Research, 34*(3), 604–612.

Tomasello, M. (1992). *First verbs: A case study of early grammatical development.* New York: Cambridge University Press.

Tomasello, M., & Farrar, J. (1986). Joint attention and early language. *Child Development, 57,* 1454–1463.

Tomasello, M., & Mervis, C.B. (1994). The instrument is great, but measuring comprehension is still a problem. In L. Fenson, P. Dale, J.S. Reznick, E. Bates, D. Thal, & S. Pethick (Eds.), Variability in early communicative development. *Monographs of the Society for Research in Child Development, 59*(5, Serial No. 242).

Truex, N.W. (1982). *An interactive concept of language development with reference to Spanish.* Unpublished doctoral dissertation, University of California, Los Angeles.

Umbel, V.M., Pearson, B.Z., Fernandez, M.C., & Oller, D.K. (1992). Measuring bilingual children's receptive vocabularies. *Child Development, 63,* 1012–1020.

van Kleeck, A., & Richardson, A. (1990). Assessment of speech and language development. In J.H. Johnson & J. Goldman (Eds.), *Developmental assessment in clinical child psychology* (pp. 132–172). New York: Pergamon Press.

Walker, D., Greenwood, C., Hart, B., & Carta, J. (1994). Prediction of school outcomes based on early language production and socioeconomic factors. *Child Development, 65,* 606–621.

Willis, S., & Edwards, J. (1996). A prelingually deaf child's acquisition of spoken vocabulary in the first year of multichannel cochlear implant use. *Child Language Teaching and Therapy, 12*(3), 272–287.

Yoder, P.J., Warren, S.F., & Biggar, H.A. (1997). Stability of maternal reports of lexical comprehension in very young children with developmental delays. *American Journal of Speech-Language Pathology, 6*(1), 59–64.

Yoder, P.J., Warren, S.F., & McCathren, R.B. (1998). Determining spoken language prognosis in children with developmental disabilities. *American Journal of Speech-Language Pathology, 7*(4), 77–87.

Zimmerman, I.L., Steiner, V.G., & Pond, R.E. (1979). *Preschool Language Scale (PLS).* San Antonio, TX: Harcourt Assessment.

Zimmerman, I.L., Steiner, V.G., & Pond, R.E. (1992). *Preschool Language Scale, Third Edition (PLS-3).* San Antonio, TX: Harcourt Assessment.

Zimmerman, I.L., Steiner, V.G., & Pond, R.E. (2002). *Preschool Language Scale, Fourth Edition (PLS-4) English edition.* San Antonio, TX: Harcourt Assessment.

Zukow, P.G. (1984). Folk theories of comprehension and caregiver style in a rural population in Central Mexico. *Quarterly Newsletter of the Laboratory of Comparative Human Cognition, 6,* 62–67.

A

BASIC INFORMATION FORM USED IN ORIGINAL NORMATIVE STUDY

BASIC INFORMATION FORM

Today's Date _____   Child's Birthdate _____

Child's Name _____   Sex _____
            FIRST   LAST

Address _____   Telephone _____

Child's Birth Order: 1st   2nd   Other _____ (*specify*)   Number of children in family _____

EXPOSURE TO OTHER LANGUAGES

Is your child regularly exposed to a language other than English?   ☐ Yes   ☐ No

If yes:

(a) What Language? _____ (b) By whom? _____ (c) How many days per week? _____
(d) How many hours per day? _____ (e) Since what age (in months)? _____

HEALTH

Has your child had any major health or speech problems?   ☐ Yes   ☐ No

If Yes, please describe.

_____

PARENT DATA

Name of parent completing form:

_____
FIRST   LAST

- -

The remaining questions are included so that we will be able to compare our sample to U.S. Census averages, not to obtain information about individual participants

OCCUPATION

Please give a specific description (e.g., computer technician, shop foreman, dental assistant, fast food manager) rather than a general category (e.g., U.S. Navy, medical field, owner, self-employed).

Mother _____
              OCCUPATION

_____
              BRIEF DESCRIPTION

Father _____
              OCCUPATION

_____
              BRIEF DESCRIPTION

EDUCATION

Please circle the highest grade completed. Use 12 for high school graduate, 16 for college graduate, and 18 for advanced degree.

Mother	6	7	8	9	10	11	12	13	14	15	16	17	18
Father	6	7	8	9	10	11	12	13	14	15	16	17	18

ETHNIC BACKGROUND

Please specify ethnic background (e.g., Asian, Black, Hispanic, White, or applicable category).

_____   _____
             MOTHER   FATHER

B

EXPANDED BASIC INFORMATION FORM

Basic Information Form

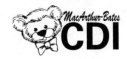

ID number _____ Today's date _____ Child's birth date _____

Child's name _____ Gender _____
        FIRST   MIDDLE   LAST

Address _____ Telephone (___)_____
        STREET   CITY   STATE   ZIP

Child's birth order ☐ 1st ☐ 2nd ☐ Other (specify) _____ Number of children in family _____

Is child adopted? ☐ yes ☐ no   Child's birth weight _____

Name of mother/guardian _____
                        FIRST   LAST

Name of father/guardian _____
                        FIRST   LAST

HEALTH

Did you experience any major
pregnancy or birth complications?   ☐ yes   ☐ no

   If yes, please describe _____

Was your child born *prematurely*
(i.e., before the due date)?   ☐ yes   ☐ no

   If yes, how many weeks early? _____

Does your child experience
chronic ear infections (5 or more)?   ☐ yes   ☐ no

   If yes, has your child undergone
   intervention (e.g., tube insertion)?   ☐ yes   ☐ no

   If yes, please describe _____

Is there some reason to suspect
that your child may have a *hearing loss?*   ☐ yes   ☐ no

Has your child had any *major illnesses,*
hospitalizations, or diagnosed disabilities?   ☐ yes   ☐ no

   If yes, please describe _____

Have *you or any member of your extended family*
(e.g., child's siblings, grandmother, father)
been diagnosed with any behavioral impairment,
neurological impairment, or language or learning disability?   ☐ yes   ☐ no

   If yes, please describe _____

Do you have *any concerns about*
your child's speech and/or language?   ☐ yes   ☐ no

   If yes, please describe _____

EXPOSURE TO OTHER LANGUAGES

Is your child *regularly exposed to*
a language(s) other than English?   ☐ yes   ☐ no

   If yes: What language(s)? _____ By whom? _____

   Number of days per week? _____ Number of hours per day? _____ Since what age (in months)? ____

Basic Information Form *(continued)*

CAREGIVER INFORMATION
With whom does your child live?

☐ One parent   ☐ Both biological parents   ☐ Biological parent and stepparent

☐ Adoptive parent(s)   ☐ Other, please explain _____

Who participates in the day-to-day care of your child?
(Check all that apply.)

☐ Mother/guardian   ☐ Child care center (_____ hours/week)

☐ Father/guardian   ☐ Non-parent caregiver (e.g., grandparent, nanny) in *your* home (_____ hours/week)

☐ Outside-the-home caregiver (e.g., family provider in that person's home) (_____ hours/week)

☐ Other (please explain) _____ (_____ hours/week)

ETHNIC BACKGROUND
Please specify your ethnic background (e.g., Asian, Black, Caucasian, Hispanic, Native American, other ethnic group).

_____   _____
         Mother/guardian   Father/guardian

EDUCATION
Please circle the highest grade completed
(12 = high school graduate, 16 = college graduate, 18 = advanced degree).

Mother/guardian: 0 1 2 3 4 5 6 7 8 9 10 11 12 13 14 15 16 17 18

Father/guardian: 0 1 2 3 4 5 6 7 8 9 10 11 12 13 14 15 16 17 18

OCCUPATION
Please provide a brief description of your *occupation* using specific terms
(e.g., computer technician, accountant, dental assistant).

Mother/guardian _____

Father/guardian _____

Approximate annual family income ($) _____

CONTACT INFORMATION
Name of parent or guardian competing this form _____

The best *time* to contact me is _____

The best *place* to contact me is   ☐ Home   Telephone _____

                                  ☐ Work   Telephone _____

Thank you for taking the time to answer our questions!
Please contact us if you have any questions or concerns.

MacArthur-Bates Communicative Development Inventories: User's Guide and Technical Manual, Second Edition, by Larry Fenson et al.
Copyright © 2007 The CDI Advisory Board. All rights reserved.
Available through Paul H. Brookes Publishing Co. • 1-800-638-3775 • 410-337-9580 • www.brookespublishing.com

C

CHILD REPORT FORMS

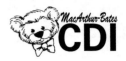

Child Report Form
CDI: Words and Gestures

ID number _____ Date of report _____ Date CDI completed _____

Child's name _____ Child's birth date _____
FIRST   MIDDLE   LAST

Parent/guardian _____ Gender _____ Child's age in months _____
FIRST   LAST

PART I: EARLY WORDS

First Signs of Understanding

Percentage of *yes* answers at this child's age (see Table 4.6)

Responds when name is called: ☐ yes ☐ no _____

Responds to "no no": ☐ yes ☐ no _____

Responds to "there's mommy/daddy": ☐ yes ☐ no _____

Phrases Understood: Number: _____ (of 28) Percentile: _____

Starting to Talk

Percentage of affirmative answers at this child's age (see Table 4.9)

Imitation: ☐ yes ☐ no _____

Labeling: ☐ yes ☐ no _____

Vocabulary Checklist

Words Understood: Number: _____ (of 396) Percentile: _____

Words Produced: Number: _____ (of 396) Percentile: _____

PART II: ACTIONS AND GESTURES

Early Gestures (Sections A and B) Number: _____ (of 18) Percentile: _____

Later Gestures (Sections C through E) Number: _____ (of 45) Percentile: _____

Total Gestures (Sections A through E) Number: _____ (of 63) Percentile: _____

Child Report Form
CDI: Words and Sentences

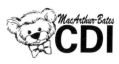

ID number _____   Date of report _____   Date CDI completed _____

Child's name _____   Child's birth date _____
FIRST   MIDDLE   LAST

Parent/guardian _____   Gender _____   Child's age in months _____
FIRST   LAST

PART I: WORDS CHILDREN USE

Vocabulary Checklist

Words Produced: Number: _____ (of 680)   Percentile: _____

How Children Use Words

Percentage of affirmative answers at this child's age (see Table 4.20)

Past:	☐ yes	☐ no	_____
Future:	☐ yes	☐ no	_____
Absent Object (Production):	☐ yes	☐ no	_____
Absent Object (Comprehension):	☐ yes	☐ no	_____
Absent Owner:	☐ yes	☐ no	_____

PART II: SENTENCES AND GRAMMAR

Word Endings/Part 1

Percentage of affirmative answers at this child's age (see Table 4.21)

Plural (-*s*):	☐ yes	☐ no	_____
Possessive (-'*s*):	☐ yes	☐ no	_____
Progressive (-*ing*):	☐ yes	☐ no	_____
Past tense (-*ed*):	☐ yes	☐ no	_____

Word Forms   Number: _____ (of 25)   Percentile: _____

Word Endings/Part 2   Number: _____ (of 45)

Combining   ☐ yes   ☐ no

Percentage of affirmative answers at this child's age (see Table 4.24)

_____

Examples

Length in morphemes of child's three longest sentences (M3L):   1. _____   2. _____   3. _____

M3L (mean): _____   Percentile: _____

Complexity

Number of times the more complex sentence is selected: _____ (of 37)   Percentile: _____

INDEX

Page numbers followed by *t* and *f* indicate tables and figures, respectively.